Stan Rodski is a highly respected scientist and an authority on how to improve mental performance in high-stress situations by adopting brain-energy management techniques. A cognitive neuroscientist, he practised as a registered psychologist for more than thirty years but now focuses on research, lecturing and writing. He currently works as a peak-performance neuroscientist and wellness expert across Australia and internationally, developing innovative technologies and programs for individuals (brain coaching), peak-performance sport and esport teams, and many top-500 companies looking for creative, brain-focused initiatives to facilitate corporate success. Most recently, he has been applying his research in the brain sciences to issues such as reducing sleep deprivation, brain fatigue and congestion, and managing and boosting energy to harness stress.

Stan introduced the brain-science-based *Colourtation* method to stress management, and his work using colouring-in techniques led to his bestselling books *Anti-stress*, *Brain-science* and *Modern Medi-tation*, which were featured in Oprah Winfrey's 2016 Christmas Wish List.

Stan's other specialist area of research is the neuroscience of machine learning – or AI (artificial intelligence) – especially using neurologically based predictive algorithms (computational neuroscience) in areas such as diversity and recruitment. Most recently, he has developed innovative 'brain-edge' scans and 'neuro-POD' technologies, which seek to revolutionise human performance in personal, learning and workplace environments.

Stan is married with four children and three grandchildren, and lives in Melbourne.

THE
NEUROSCIENCE
OF
EXCELLENT
SLEEP

THE
NEUROSCIENCE
OF
EXCELLENT
SLEEP

HOW NEUROSCIENCE AND MINDFULNESS CAN
HELP YOU GET A GOOD NIGHT'S SLEEP, WORK
MORE EFFICIENTLY AND LEAD A HEALTHIER LIFE

STAN RODSKI

HarperCollins*Publishers*

HarperCollins*Publishers*
Australia • Brazil • Canada • France • Germany • Holland • India
Italy • Japan • Mexico • New Zealand • Poland • Spain • Sweden
Switzerland • United Kingdom • United States of America

HarperCollins acknowledges the Traditional Custodians of the land upon
which we live and work, and pays respect to Elders past and present.

First published in Australia in 2023
by HarperCollins*Publishers* Australia Pty Limited
Gadigal Country
Level 13, 201 Elizabeth Street, Sydney NSW 2000
ABN 36 009 913 517
harpercollins.com.au

A catalogue record for this book is available from the National Library
of Australia

ISBN 978 1 4607 5382 8 (paperback)
ISBN 978 1 4607 0832 3 (ebook)
ISBN 978 1 4607 8120 3 (audiobook)

Cover design: Design by Committee
Cover and internal images by shutterstock.com
Design and layout by Jude Rowe

To my three precious and beautiful grandchildren,
Ellie Rodski, Harry Rodski and Tex Alexander

CONTENTS

LIGHTS ON: LET'S TALK ABOUT SLEEP

*'There is a time for many words,
and there is also a time for sleep'*

—Homer

Our brain operates continuously, day and night, for every day of our lives. As it goes about its twenty-four-hour cycle, it switches functions to accommodate our changing needs – and one of the most important of those needs is sleep. It's an activity that occupies about one-third of our lives. For many of us, it feels quite simple. When we get tired, we shuffle off to bed and go to sleep for the next seven to eight hours (or for some of us considerably less than that). But in many ways its purposes remain a mystery to us. And the more that neuroscience – the study of the brain – uncovers, the more scientists have come to understand just how complicated a process it is.

Over the past five years I've lectured on sleep to students and staff at many universities on behalf of a major health insurer. You might ask – quite reasonably – why would an insurance company invest so heavily in an area like sleep? The answer is a simple one: better sleep strongly correlates with better health, and better health means better business. The health effects not just of illnesses such as insomnia and sleep apnoea but also of poor or insufficient sleep are front and centre in the minds of the insurers, and increasingly in the minds of the rest of us.

In my lectures, one of my young students will almost inevitably explain away their constant studying and partying with the words: 'Plenty of time to sleep when I'm dead.' I hear similar things from hardworking executives, who claim that they'll get all the sleep they need when they finally shuffle off this mortal coil we call life.

Ironically, death may catch up with all of these people far more quickly than they think. Put simply, extreme lack of sleep can kill, as chronic fatigue increases our risk of disease, illness and early mortality.

Both these groups have failed to understand the true significance of sleep. As far as they're concerned, it's not

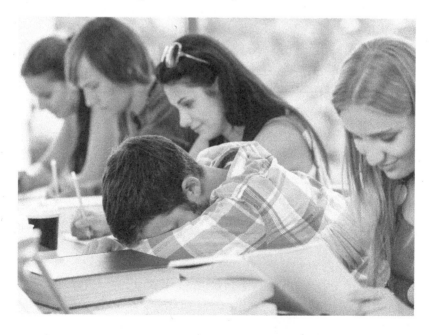

something that needs to be focused on, let alone something that could be improved, even to the point of excellence. Why do so many of us have an acute awareness of other aspects of our health, but see sleep as something that 'just happens'?

In this book I want to convince you that sleep is an essential pillar of good health and needs to be taken seriously and prioritised. I want to show you what happens when sleep is done right, and what can occur when it goes wrong. And I want to explain why. I want to persuade you that adequate sleep is essential for the health of our entire body and brain, and that we require both sleep *quantity* and sleep *quality*. Excellent sleep occurs when we get both.

But what about those of us who would *desperately love* to get those seven to eight hours' sleep a night, but can't? Maybe you suffer from a health complaint or sleep disorder, maybe your job means you sleep irregular hours, or perhaps you just can't stop thinking about the events of the day when you turn out the lights at night.

Sleep and relaxation are so important to our overall wellbeing, but increasingly difficult to achieve in our digitally based, fast-paced, time-poor and stress-filled world. A book like this can't provide answers for all the problems associated with sleep, but the brain-based exercises included here will relieve most symptoms of poor sleep and leave you feeling calm and relaxed.

If you have trouble sleeping and have kids, you're probably keen to set them up to be far better sleepers than you. We all want to do what's best for our children, even if this means less sleep for ourselves. My interest in the sleep needs of children – from babies to adolescents – began forty-two years ago, with the birth of my first child. An infant can present many challenges when it comes to sleeping, not just for the child, but also for the adults who are trying to care for and nurture them. Working in an executive health practice for

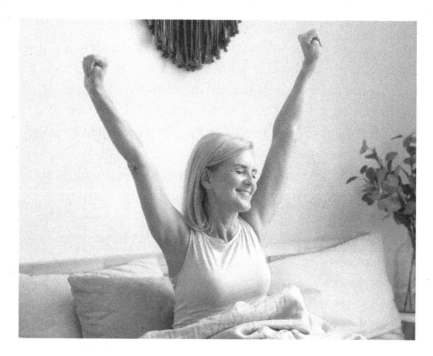

fifteen years revealed to me that many people's sleep issues were very much tied up with problems their children were having with sleep.

When our children sleep at odd hours, or wake in the night with sleep terrors, it's tempting to assume that they're naturally poor sleepers – just as we do when we can't sleep ourselves. But the great news is that, regardless of our current sleep patterns, nearly all of us have an inherent ability to fall asleep and remain asleep. Like most adults, virtually all children have the ability to achieve good, even *excellent* sleep.

For the vast majority of us, sleep is something we don't think about until we have to. But ask anybody, 'How was your sleep last night?' and the answer is almost always: 'It could have been better.'

So why not work on *making* it better? Why not work towards being able to say, 'I had an *excellent* sleep'?

If we start to look at sleep as a twenty-four-hour process, and not just a waste of seven to eight hours, we can then begin to link the activities of our wakeful periods to our sleep periods and give ourselves a real chance of achieving an *excellent sleep.*

Time to turn the lights on so we can take a good look at how to do just that.

Why not work towards being able to say,
'I had an excellent sleep'?

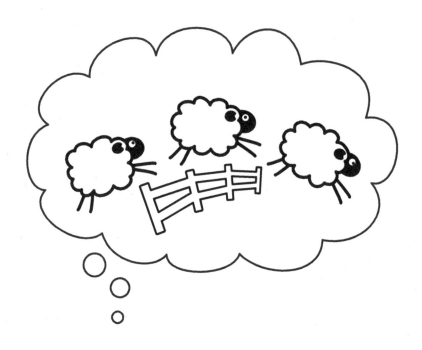

PART 1

WHY WE NEED TO SLEEP

'Let her sleep, for when she wakes, she will shake the world.'

—Napoleon Bonaparte,
French general and emperor (1769–1821)

THE PURPOSE OF SLEEP

How sleep happens, and what's going on while it happens, are complex questions, and yet at face value very simple. Sleep literally involves doing nothing but lying down and not being conscious.

The purpose of sleep is a very hot topic, widely debated among scientists. Clearly, sleep is for **rest**, which allows our body and brain time to recover and recharge. Periods of activity that leave us feeling exhausted need to be followed by prolonged periods of inactivity to give our system time to recover and be replenished.

But sleeping is not just resting. The amount of sleep we need is not dependent on the amount of activity we've engaged in. We can usually sleep around seven hours whether we have completed hard manual labour or lain around on the lounge all day. One activity requires recuperation and the other does not, which is why exhaustion does not dictate our sleep patterns. As we'll see, the timing and duration of our sleep are determined not by our need to rest but by our body's **circadian rhythm**, our biological clock.

Our **body temperature** drops by 1 or 2 degrees during sleep, which suggests that sleep is about more than just resting and conserving energy. When animals hibernate, both their metabolism and their temperature drop to an almost comatose state, during which they move in and out of sleep. This process uses an enormous amount of energy and confirms just how complicated sleep is. Seeing it as simply about resting and re-energising is very much underestimating sleep.

Sleep's role in **physical healing** and **defusing negative emotions** is well documented. But more recently, scientific theories have focused on sleep's ability to remove weak neurological connections and **improve brain function**.

Sleep and brain performance

Believe it or not, sleep can actually help us become more intelligent and develop better problem-solving and decision-making skills, reasoning and judgment.

The act of learning involves a highly efficient ability to remember information. If we learn something before going to sleep, or even having a nap, the brain replays that information many times while we sleep. We'll wake up remembering it better than before we went to bed.

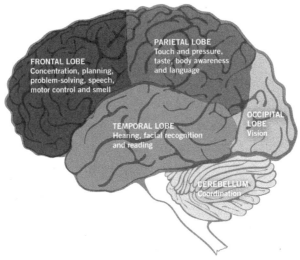

Major functions of the brain

The process begins when we take information that we captured with our five senses, then temporarily store it in our brain's memory-holding tank, called the **hippocampus** (page 56). (We'll learn more about the different parts of the brain in **Part 2**.)

Processing this information requires us to transfer it to the outer layer of the brain, the **cortex** (page 55). The cortex then proceeds to consolidate (choose what is important and discard what is not), edit (rearrange and restructure), and file what we've learned into our long-term memory until we need to retrieve it again. This is called **long-term potentiation**. Connections between relevant neurons (nerve cells) are strengthened, including memories. Meanwhile, to avoid overactivity and optimise energy use, less important connections are weakened or removed. This means that when we are awake, significant connections will become stronger.

Our old memories must be connected to our new ones to help reinforce learning and, most importantly, improve accessibility. Our very old memories regularly need to be stimulated, so that the connections, and the memories attached to them, are not lost. This same process also takes place when we develop new skills. It goes on during sleep because it's the most efficient time for the brain to do it. There are no distractions, and no new information is demanding attention.

It's been found that different types of memories are consolidated during different stages of sleep. If we wake in the second half of the night, when most of our **dream sleep** occurs, we don't consolidate learned motor skills. If we wake early in the night, we may lose our verbal learning.

During **deep sleep**, our brain is actively carrying out the task of converting fresh experiences into long-term memories. In dream sleep, an area of the brain called the **associative cortex** is particularly active. This allows us to come up with new and useful ideas, link concepts and thoughts in novel ways, or simply tap into our creative process. Our brain continues to work on problems that baffle us, and it may come up with the right answer only after we've rested. Only in the dream phase of sleep is our brain capable of carrying out this process, and it's mostly during this stage that our brain reinforces, organises and maintains our 'memory files'.

Sleep also provides an opportunity for the brain to remove information and a wide variety of by-products that it *doesn't* need. The complex ongoing cellular activity of the brain produces material that needs to be treated as waste and removed. While this occurs all the time, during sleep the brain is particularly active in its waste management.

Dreaming

What exactly is dreaming? That's a very difficult question for scientists to answer, because records of dreams are almost entirely dependent on self-reporting. We usually don't remember our dreams and, when we do, our memories are normally very sketchy. Those memories don't provide the scientific rigour required for real understanding.

Having said that, two prevailing theories are subject to ongoing research. The first of these is the **activation–synthesis theory** and the second is the **clinico-anatomical theory**.

The activation–synthesis theory focuses on the brain's attempt to make sense of distorted and scant information. At the beginning of a dream, the brain's **pons** region (page 39) is activated and, in turn, waves generated by the pons activate parts of the cortex. This frenetic activation is combined in the cortex with any other activity under way and is fused into something more rational and meaningful. Our brain temporarily stores information that evokes emotion in a structure called the **amygdala** (page 55). Because the pons and the amygdala work together, our dreams often have emotions attached to them. (We'll learn more about how activity in the pons region contributes to dreaming when we look at *Stage 5 sleep* in **Part 2** [page 39]).

The clinico-anatomical theory defines dreams as a form of thinking occurring in unusual conditions. This theory contends that the activity of our sensory organs – our vision, hearing, smell, taste and touch – is reduced, vision and hearing in particular. Because the **motor cortex** – which controls our body's movement – is dormant, no actions can occur. The **prefrontal cortex** is also dormant, meaning our working (recent) memory is impeded and we will be unable to remember the dream and what went on in it.

With these parts of the brain shut down, other areas are able to create images without restriction. The upper regions of the **visual cortex** become busy creating the vivid pictures we often associate with our dreams. The amygdala is also busy adding emotions. Activation of these brain areas, combined with no actual sensory input, is thought to create the hallucinations we call dreams.

We know that in dream sleep, the higher, more sophisticated centres of the brain receive stimulation from deeper, more primitive brain regions. Impulses come up the same sensory pathways that are used for sights, sounds and perhaps touch, smell and taste. It is thought that these stimuli are incorporated by the brain into dream imagery.

The purpose of dreams

While the content of our dreams is unpredictable, they do tend to occur when we have something on our mind, particularly a difficult issue. We'll tend to think about the issue during our waking hours, which causes the brain to seek ways to organise these thoughts, usually in our dreams, where solutions may be found. Unfortunately these solutions are often impractical, but they can create a path for us to think further about the issue when we wake.

On the other side of the coin, the activation and maintenance of memories cause them to be effectively rehashed in our brain. Very old experiences and more recent imaginings are all thrown into the mix together. There is no specific order or logical structure to the sequence of experiences this results in. This is why dreams are so otherworldly and bizarre.

One theory is that the frontal regions of the brain responsible for attention and logic are trying to impose some sort of rationale on this ramshackle sequence of events, which explains why we still feel as if dreams are real while they're happening, and the impossible occurrences don't strike us as unusual when we're dreaming.

Sleep provides an opportunity for the brain to remove information and a wide variety of by-products that it doesn't need.

WHEN SLEEP GOES WRONG

When sleep goes *right*, our brain is successfully acquiring new information and finding creative solutions through our dreams. When sleep goes *wrong* – either we don't get enough, or it's poor in quality – there can be a whole array of consequences, both short- and long-term.

How much sleep do I need?

Our sleep requirements vary considerably throughout our lifetime. Although there is no magic number of hours that guarantees a satisfying slumber, the graph opposite is a good general guide to sleep needs across our lifespan.

As it shows, sleep is especially important to children as they rapidly acquire and reinforce learned information. Infants sleep more than half the day, with extended periods of dream sleep, to optimise brain efficiency. Our sleep needs tail off as we reach adolescence, then are further reduced in the final few decades of life.

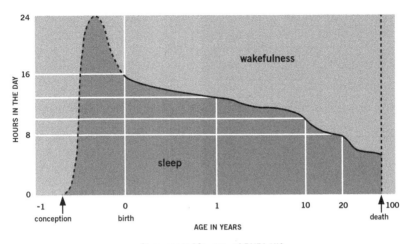

Sleep needs (*Courtesy of BUPA UK*)

Depending on your age, here is the number of hours' sleep you should aim for each night, according to the science from multiple medical fields.

Age in Years	Recommended Hours of Sleep
0–1	14–15
1–3	12–14
3–6	10–12
7–12	10–11
12–25	8–9
26–64	7–9
65+	7–8

We've just been looking at how important sleep is for our brain and body. In spite of this, quite a few people skimp on sleep hours and try to get by with the least number possible. Studies suggest that many adults 'survive' on less than six hours' sleep per night, possibly less if they have electronic devices in the bedroom that go off and interrupt their sleep cycle.

Sometimes this may be due to misinformation about sleep. More often than not, the students I talked about in my introduction believed they slept as much as they needed to: sometimes as little as four hours. The reality is that four hours are not nearly enough for an *excellent sleep*. Sleeping so little on a regular basis will in fact impair not just their immediate performance but also their longer-term health and wellbeing.

Excellent sleep is about not only the *quantity* of sleep but also the *quality*. It's not just that many people aren't getting *enough* sleep, it's also that their sleep is often punctuated by **wakefulness**. Over time, lack of quality sleep can lead to chronic health problems, or cause chronic problems to worsen.

Lost sleep

As we've just seen, most of us adults need at least seven or eight hours of sleep per night. Few of us can get by with as little as three or four hours a night without apparent side effects.

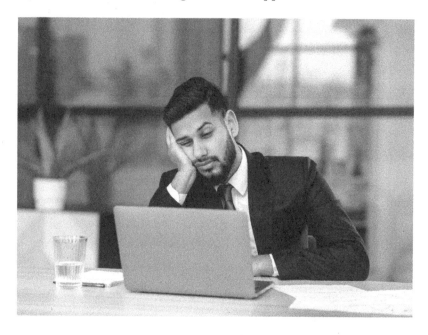

We're all familiar with the consequences of lost sleep. (They're probably why most of us are reading this book.) We may feel groggy and irritable. Our focus is probably off and we don't perform at our best. We're likely to dump sugary foods into our system for an energy boost. Or we'll try to use coffee, or other stimulants such as energy drinks, to improve our alertness. (The caffeine in coffee does this by blocking the receptors for **adenosine**, a chemical that increases drowsiness.)

The longer we're awake, the more our alertness diminishes. The release of the brain's primary inhibitor, called **GABA** (gamma aminobutyric acid), increases while we sleep and accumulates in our neurons when we are deprived of sleep. The increase in GABA gradually impairs our concentration, so that our attention lapses and we fail to notice important things around us.

When we're getting enough sleep, we tend to notice these lapses and jump back into a more aroused state. When we are sleep-deprived we tend not to notice. If we go too long without sleep, our brain starts to initiate sleep whether we want it or not, causing micro-sleeps for between a second and a minute at a time. The brain is trying to grab some small crumbs of sleep, which are inadequate, because our brain needs long periods of unconsciousness. Lack of sleep also greatly reduces our motor skills and reaction time. All of this is particularly dangerous if we are driving a car or doing some kind of risky activity.

One of the most important effects of sleeplessness is on our memory. If we are sleep-deprived, we greatly diminish our ability to capture, store and retrieve information. Quite simply, we cannot think effectively.

Lack of sleep may also cause our brain's **prefrontal cortex** – which normally keeps our emotional responses in check – to shut down. This can lead us to overreact to negative experiences. Instead of facing our problems like a well-reasoned adult, we'll be more apt to speak and act with moodiness, impatience and irritation when the stress hormones come into play. A major part of my work as a psychologist and neuroscientist focuses on how stress can create a vicious cycle: stress releases a hormone called cortisol, which interferes with sleep patterns and results in yet more stress (more on this later).

But the effects of sleep deprivation go way beyond these concerns. So what are some of the *more serious* implications of poor sleep?

Health problems

Sleep plays a significant role in managing levels of stress, obesity, blood sugar, inflammation, hormones, immunity and depression. Consequently, **sleep deprivation** has a broad array of connections with poor health. Chronic lack of sleep can cause, contribute to and co-exist with many major illnesses and chronic diseases, and therefore increase our risk of dying prematurely.

So, as I say to my students in the sleep class, this may be the only lecture they attend where falling asleep is quite OK.

Heart health

Lack of sleep has been found to contribute to hypertension, or high blood pressure, by keeping the nervous system in a state of hyperactivity. High blood pressure in turn affects the heart and blood vessels throughout the body. In one study, each hour of lost sleep was associated with a 35 per cent higher chance of developing hypertension. Merely shutting our eyes, turning out the lights and lying face up can produce a significant drop in blood pressure.

People with sleep problems have been found to have higher levels of molecules such as cytokines, which trigger inflammation and can, in turn, make such people more susceptible to serious inflammatory diseases, including cancers. They may also have higher levels of fibrinogen – a protein that is responsible for blood-clotting – together with a faster heart rate. This kind of inflammation, and the resulting plaque build-up in arteries, may be due to the large amount of the aforementioned stress hormone cortisol that is released when sleep is poor.

Generally, people who have trouble falling asleep may be as much as 70 per cent more likely to have a coronary event.

Weight gain and obesity

When we sleep less than six hours a night, we are more likely to gain weight and have an increase in body fat and a bigger waist circumference. Research has found that those who sleep less than four hours nightly have a 73 per cent chance of becoming obese, whereas those who sleep six hours have a 23 per cent chance of obesity. According to the National Sleep

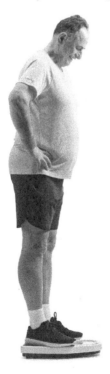

Foundation in the United States, 77 per cent of obese adults report some kind of sleep problem. This may help to explain why university students, shift workers, new parents and others who are sleep-poor often put on extra kilos.

Scientists are not certain why they occur, but some interesting chemical changes have been observed in those who experience sleep loss. The levels of the appetite-suppressing hormone **leptin** fall, while levels of the appetite-stimulating hormone **ghrelin** rise. These hormonal changes are associated with greater hunger and stronger cravings for carbohydrates.

There is a close association between stress, obesity, **type 2 diabetes** and inflammation. Each has a significant influence over the others. Experts have noted that a lack of sleep lowers our insulin resistance and increases our risk of type 2 diabetes, because it impairs the body's ability to regulate blood pressure. In one study, getting less than four hours of sleep nightly for only one week was enough to disrupt the way people's bodies processed carbohydrates. Metabolic issues such as these usually result in weight gain.

The stress hormone cortisol is also closely associated with more abdominal fat, and the abnormally high levels of cortisol

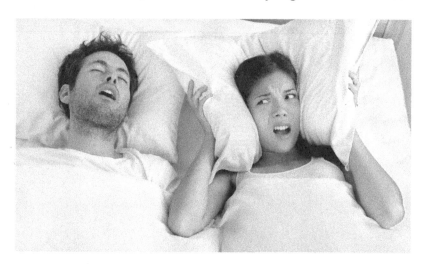

recorded in those with poor sleep can trigger weight gain. As noted, cortisol may also be a cause of inflammation.

At the same time, people who are overweight tend to have less restful sleep due to issues such as heartburn, snoring and **sleep apnoea** (page 23). This can further exacerbate weight problems, and the process can turn into a vicious cycle of its own.

Pain

Pain, particularly chronic pain, is one of the most pervasive medical conditions around the world. In the United States alone, it is estimated that one in five people are affected by conditions such as headaches, back pain and pain from arthritis, cancer and injuries. The cost to that country is estimated to be $61 billion in lost productivity and significantly more in medical costs.

According to the US National Sleep Foundation, pain is a leading cause of insomnia. Approximately 20 per cent of adults in the United States report pain that disrupts their sleep.

Pain and sleeplessness share a constellation of symptoms, including fatigue and depression. And areas of the brain involved in our perception of pain – including the **frontal cortex** and **limbic system** – are the same ones involved in falling asleep and staying asleep. So experiencing pain causes sleeplessness, and poor-quality sleep makes pain worse. For example, a person with lower back pain may become aroused from sleep several times per hour. Being sleep-deprived will leave that person less able to cope with the pain the next day.

Fibromyalgia

This is a condition affecting significant numbers of people worldwide. Sufferers experience widespread pain and tenderness in their muscles, bones and soft tissues, leading to a general sense of fatigue. Data from the US alone estimates that fibromyalgia affects 10 million people. It has no obvious bodily causes and does not show up on X-rays.

Growing evidence suggests that fibromyalgia is partly a brain disorder that throws our pain pathways into disarray so that the brain responds to imaginary wounds. The natural opioid system that regulates pain perception becomes dysfunctional. Disrupted sleep only worsens the chronic pain.

Fibromyalgia is associated with low levels of **serotonin**, a chemical produced during the deepest stage of sleep. The fact that women produce lower levels of serotonin may help explain why more than 90 per cent of people with fibromyalgia are female.

Dysfunction of the serotonin pathway affects the person's perception of pain. Serotonin influences the pain threshold by interacting with **substance P**, a chemical that sends information about tissue injury and damage from receptors in the body to the brain. Levels of substance P are higher in people with fibromyalgia. It builds up in the body's tissues and eventually transmits painful impulses to the spinal cord and brain, which lowers the person's pain threshold.

Any increase in pain can cause deep sleep to become disrupted, and vice versa. Even young, healthy people who have sleep disruptions can experience the kind of increases in muscle tenderness that occur in fibromyalgia. When they go back to their normal sleep patterns, their discomfort diminishes, and in most cases soon goes away completely.

Other health problems

The influence of poor sleep on memory and brain function has implications for diseases such as **Alzheimer's** and **Parkinson's**. With both illnesses, sleep disturbances may be an early symptom, long before memory or movement symptoms become apparent or are diagnosed.

Too little sleep has also been associated with **breast cancer** and **colon cancer**, which in some cases are suspected to be due to a combination of hormone levels, immune functioning and body weight. For some, lack of sleep can also contribute to **poor mental health** and increase the risk of mental illness.

Too much sleep

Some researchers have also warned that too much sleep – more than nine hours per night – can lead to inflammation, lower levels of good cholesterol, higher levels of bad cholesterol, and a greater risk of heart disease, stroke and death. It is not clear why, but it is possibly due to the fact that people who sleep longer are more likely to be depressed or chronically ill.

Sleep disorders

There is also a range of disorders specifically associated with sleep. Most of them have particular causes that need regular attention. The exercises in **Part 3** of this book may provide some relief from these conditions – and from the health problems we've just looked at – but many of the conditions will also require expert medical treatment.

Sleep apnoea

Sleep apnoea occurs when a person has trouble breathing during sleep. Sufferers experience breathless periods of about sixty seconds, which cause them to wake often, gasping for breath. The next day they frequently won't remember these periods of waking up, but will feel the effects, potentially, of all the issues we've just looked at under **Lost sleep** and **Health problems**.

The causes of sleep apnoea include ageing of brain areas that control breathing; hormones; and of course genetics. Sleep apnoea affects multiple brain areas, reducing the number of neurons, which decreases the brain's ability to control impulses and take in new information. It's not known whether these issues in the brain *cause* sleep apnoea or the other way around, but the link between the two is strong.

There is no doubt about the link between sleep apnoea and obesity, particularly for men in mid-life. Obesity causes the airway to narrow, meaning that breathing becomes both more frequent and more forceful. It is difficult to maintain this type of breathing, particularly if the airway is further obstructed by an awkward sleeping posture.

The individual sufferer can do things themselves to control sleep apnoea, such as avoid alcohol and lose weight. Others resort to medical interventions, such as surgical removal of the tissue that obstructs the trachea (breathing passage). There are also technological interventions, such as using a breathing apparatus that helps keep the airways open by delivering air under pressure.

Narcolepsy

Sufferers of narcolepsy frequently find themselves feeling sleepy and/or falling asleep during the day. Narcolepsy will look different for different sufferers. They may have sudden or gradual attacks of sleepiness in daytime. They may suffer a cataplexy, which causes their muscles to feel weak and lose control. Interestingly, cataplexy is often accompanied by strong emotions, ranging from joy to anger.

Further effects can include sleep paralysis while falling asleep or waking up, and even dreamlike experiences or hallucinations – usually experienced when falling asleep – that may be difficult to distinguish from reality.

So what is the cause of all this? The culprit is the neurotransmitter (chemical brain-messenger) **orexin**. Orexin helps keep us awake, and without it we tend to alternate between short waking periods and sleeping periods rather than staying awake all day. The brains of narcolepsy sufferers lack the **hypothalamic cells** that release orexin. The reason is unknown, but we know it's not genetic.

While no specific drug has been found to stimulate the release of orexin, narcoleptics are often prescribed Ritalin (methylphenidate) to strengthen the brain's production of **norepinephrine** and **dopamine**, chemicals that give us energy and wake us up.

Twitchy leg syndrome

This syndrome, also known as **periodic limb movement disorder**, involves repeated involuntary movement of the legs during sleep. Most of us experience an occasional involuntary movement or kick, particularly when we're falling asleep. The problem begins when this becomes persistent and affects the quality of our sleep. During non-dream sleep, the sufferer will experience leg kicks every thirty seconds or so, for anywhere from minutes to hours at a time. When the kicks are particularly violent, they can wake the sufferer and anyone near them.

Hypnic jerks

The **hypnic jerk** or **myoclonus** is another type of uncontrolled movement but, unlike twitchy leg syndrome, it occurs *while we fall asleep*. The sufferer feels as if they're falling suddenly, and finds themselves unexpectedly twitching and spasming. This condition occurs more often in children, and gradually declines as we age.

Hypnic jerks have been associated with anxiety, stress and other sleep disorders, but overall they seem to be largely random. The reasons behind them are largely unknown, but what is known is that they are harmless.

Sleep terrors, talks and walks

Sleep terrors occur during non-dream sleep when we experience intense anxiety from which we wake screaming in terror. This is very different from a nightmare, which is simply a bad or unpleasant dream, experienced mostly by children (as we'll learn in **Part 4**).

Sleep talking, on the other hand, is harmless and common in people of all ages. It occurs at all stages of sleep and its duration is extremely variable.

Sleepwalking is most common during deep sleep, early in the night. It is not completely understood, but it may be connected with the stages of sleep when our brain becomes incredibly active and the motor neurons that control body movement are switched off, to prevent us from causing injuries to ourselves. In sleepwalkers, this system may not be working because it is not powerful enough or lacks enough coordination. This 'tangling' of the brain's control system reflects just how active our brain is when we sleep.

Only 1 per cent of adults are sleepwalkers. As we'll see in **Part 4**, sleepwalking is more common in children, usually when they are sleep-deprived. Scientists suggest that this is because their motor inhibition systems are not yet fully developed. Some studies point to underdevelopment of the central nervous system as a likely cause, or at least a contributing factor.

Sleepwalking is more common in certain families, suggesting that this immaturity of the central nervous system may be partly genetic. But it can also occur in adults under the influence of such factors as stress, alcohol, drugs and medication, all of which might also affect this motor inhibition system.

Sleep paralysis

Sleep paralysis is another condition where the brain forgets to switch the motor functions back on as we regain our consciousness, with the result that the sufferer cannot move his or her body. It may be because of disruptions as we pass through the various sleep cycles during the night. If the transition between one stage and the next happens too quickly, with too much strength, or for too long, we will wake up without proper motor control.

The sleep paralysis is usually short-lived, and our brain soon becomes alert so we can resume normal functioning. Still, we can be left feeling helpless and vulnerable. This paralysis has been known to trigger hallucinations involving danger, and a strong sense that there is another person in the room.

For most of us these are rare occurrences, but for a small few, sleep paralysis can become a chronic, persistent concern. Those who experience the brain-processing issues of sleep paralysis often suffer from depression too. It's not clear whether the depression is a result of this terrifying event or the other way round.

Insomnia

All of the above disorders are forms of sleeplessness, or insomnia. Not all of us who are sleep-deprived are insomniacs, though. My sleep students, flat out partying and studying; executives busy climbing the corporate ladder – these groups are deliberately depriving themselves of sleep. Others, such as parents of a crying baby, are being kept awake for other reasons they can't control. But what if you lie in bed for seven to eight hours, with no outside disturbances, and just aren't getting enough sleep? Maybe you can't drift off

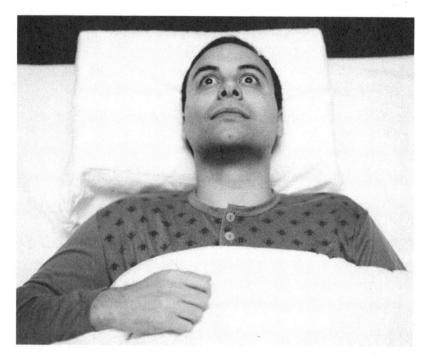

when you first go to bed; maybe you wake in the middle of the night and can't get back to sleep; or maybe you wake early in the morning and just lie there till it's time to get up. If this is you, you're suffering from either acute (short-term) or chronic (long-term) insomnia.

We've already met a series of disorders with specific causes, but general insomnia can have a range of causes too. These include stress, pain, diet, noise, medications and temperature. As we've seen, it can also result from many medical conditions, and can frequently make those conditions even worse.

Of course, many of these problems require medical intervention that is beyond the scope of this book. But there's a lot we can do *ourselves* to relieve the symptoms of insomnia. As we'll see in **Part 3**, by embracing the principles of neuroscience we can learn to relax our brain and body with short, simple exercises that can be done at any time of the day, or in some cases before or after bed. And the great news is that for a lot of us, if we put in the work, it may be enough to reduce or even eliminate our insomnia, which will set us on the path to good, even *excellent* sleep.

But first, we'll need to know a lot more about what actually happens when we sleep. In **Part 2**, we're going to learn about the different stages of sleep we pass through each night, about our biological clock – and other types of insomnia affected by it – and about the effect of sleep on our body temperature and emotions. This will help us understand what is waking us up. Then we'll look at what we can do about it to help ourselves (**Part 3**) and our children (**Part 4**).

There's a lot we can do ourselves to relieve the symptoms of insomnia and set us on the path to excellent sleep.

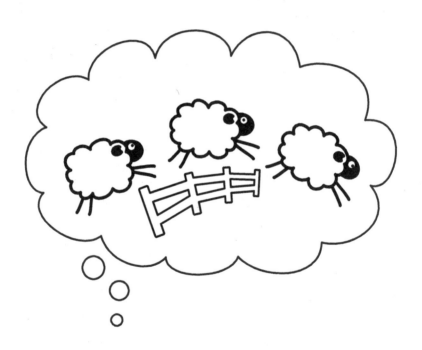

PART 2

WHAT HAPPENS WHEN WE SLEEP

'Each night when I go to sleep, I die.
And the next morning, when I wake up,
I'm reborn.'

—Mahatma Gandhi,
Indian activist and leader (1869–1948)

THE STAGES OF SLEEP

Much of what goes on while we're asleep remains a mystery to us. We may look at the clock at 11pm, and the next thing we know it's 7am, and all we can remember of those eight hours is a few dreams and perhaps a trip to the bathroom.

Nonetheless, our brain isn't simply turned off like an unplugged computer. Chemical reactions are generating constant electrical activity, which can be picked up on the surface of the scalp by sensitive electrodes. This was known as far back as the 1920s, when researchers demonstrated that an **EEG (electroencephalograph)** could detect and record this activity.

Sleep and the EEG

The EEG is a machine that records the average strength of the electrical pulses in the brain by means of a series of electrodes placed on the head. The EEG measures rises and falls of brain waves, when the cells and fibres of the brain do the same things *at the same time*.

Imagine you're recording the sound at a birthday party. It will be just noise with slight variations, until everyone starts singing at once with the entrance of the birthday cake. It is this sudden increase in 'brain noise', *in unison*, that the EEG records.

If you've ever participated in a Mexican wave at a major public event, then you've synchronised *your* wave to other people's. As different parts of our brain communicate with each other, they synchronise their patterns of activity, or **brain waves**, in the same way.

Brain waves are generated by the pulses of electrical activity our neurons produce as they communicate with each other. Our thoughts, feelings and actions are all expressed through this constant neural communication – so our brain waves are associated with how we feel and behave at any given moment.

Brain waves have been compared with the waves created when you throw stones into a pond. Toss in a single stone and a ripple of waves spreads out, becoming larger and larger. In much the same way, activity from a single cell of the brain will be captured on an EEG as a distinct wave.

Throw a handful of pebbles into the water, and what you observe is a jumbled mess. It's impossible to discern any pattern in the waves. The same thing happens when our brain is very active, with numerous sites processing information and firing. The resulting waves are small, irregular and chaotic.

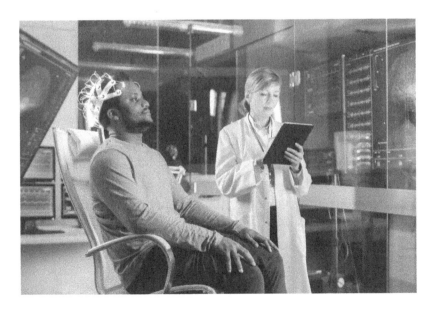

The faster (and higher in frequency) the brain-wave pattern, the greater our state of arousal. The slower and lower-frequency our brain waves are, the deeper our state of relaxation – or sleep.

Each night we go through **five stages of sleep** – four **non-REM (rapid eye movement) stages** and one **REM stage**:

1. Stage 1 (non-REM)

2. Stage 2 (non-REM)

3. Stage 3 (non-REM)

4. Stage 4 (non-REM)

5. Stage 5: REM sleep

When we're awake, and during each stage of sleep, our brain is engaged in a different type of activity, indicated by a different brain-wave frequency.

Our brain during the day

When we're awake and active, the waves our brains produce – **beta waves** – are fast and have no constant pattern. They are also high in frequency: they measure between 15 and 40 hertz (Hz), which means they oscillate (move up then down) between fifteen and forty times every second. As we move towards sleep, the amplitude (strength) of the brain waves will diminish and the frequency of the brain waves will decrease to somewhere between 8 and 12 Hz.

We can be involved in deep concentration or logical thinking, we can be watching or listening to something, or we can just be sitting quietly. We might be engaging in conversation, or performing work or exercise. This is a state of mind in which we are alert and completely aware of our circumstances. When beta brain-wave patterns dominate, we're primed to focus and concentrate, to make decisions and think analytically. The more excited we become, the higher the number of brain-wave oscillations we produce per second. At the highest levels, beta waves are associated with anxiety.

Preparing for sleep

As we close our eyes in preparation for sleep, our brain enters a stage of wakeful relaxation. We are groggy, but not yet asleep. In the EEG recording below, you can see a steady series of alpha waves. Slower than beta waves and lower in frequency (between 9 and 14 Hz), alpha waves are dominant when we're drowsy but still alert. Mindfulness, meditation and yoga all help us achieve an alpha state; it is also good for creativity. (In **Part 3**, we'll look at exercises that encourage our brain to produce these wonderful, sleep-inducing waves.)

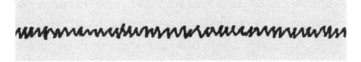

The brain while awake but with eyes closed

Stage 1 sleep

This is a state of peacefulness, rest and reflection. Our body temperature drops, our muscles relax, and we begin to lose awareness of our surroundings. But we can be easily jarred into wakefulness, and if that happens, it may be hard to distinguish whether we were just drowsy or actually asleep.

During this stage our brain waves slow down further and are interspersed with theta waves, which are slower than alpha waves and of a lower frequency (between 5 and 8 Hz). That murky barrier between sleep and wakefulness, when we're drifting in and out of sleep, and our thoughts feel dreamlike and difficult to remember? That's a theta-dominant state of consciousness.

Our brain activity is lower than during the state of wakeful relaxation, but higher than during later sleep stages. In this critical stage, as in wakefulness, the brain's cortex receives a lot of information from the hippocampus – the brain's memory-holding tank – at high frequencies. It decides what information it wishes to keep and what it will remove as 'rubbish'. The neurons are active, but not all at the same time. This produces an EEG like the one below, full of rapid, short and choppy waves.

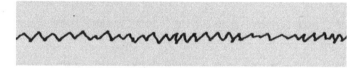

The brain during Stage 1 sleep

Stage 2 sleep

As the number of theta waves increases and our brain-wave pattern becomes more uniform, we begin Stage 2, the first stage of proper sleep. There is a slow reduction in brain activity and it is much harder for us to wake up.

However, these slower waves are interspersed with irregular bursts of fast activity called **sleep spindles**. They are high in frequency (12 to 14 Hz) and usually last around half a second. They're the result of oscillating interactions between cells in the thalamus and the cortex. About every two minutes, **K-complexes** – sudden increases in amplitude – also occur. This is part of our built-in security system, which keeps us ready to be awakened if necessary.

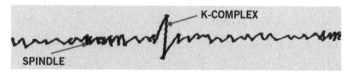

The brain during Stage 2 sleep

Research shows that sleep spindles increase in number after we've learned something new. This is consistent among most humans, on any given night of sleep. The more spindle activity, the more learning.

Stage 3 sleep

As we transition in and out of this lighter sleep state, our mind reaches a level of deeper meditation. Eventually we enter Stage 3 sleep, also known as 'slow-wave sleep' or 'restorative sleep'. Our heart rate, breathing rate and brain activity decrease. We begin to experience very slow, coordinated, large-amplitude **delta waves** that are very low in frequency (between 1.5 and 4 Hz). This is the dominant brain-wave pattern of deep, non-REM sleep (Stages 3 and 4).

In Stages 1 and 2 we can easily awaken, but in Stages 3 and 4 we become very unresponsive to the outside world and can only be aroused with difficulty. If we do wake up, we'll be disoriented and groggy. But deep sleep does not mean the brain is totally shut down, because even when it operates at this very low level, it has multiple roles in maintaining sleep and keeping our body functioning.

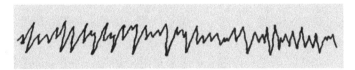

The brain during Stage 3 sleep

Stage 4 sleep

As the proportion of delta waves exceeds 50 per cent, we enter Stage 4 sleep. More than 50 per cent of those waves last for half a second or more.

Our system seems to be on autopilot. Our breathing becomes slow and regular. Our blood pressure and pulse fall to 20 per cent below waking levels.

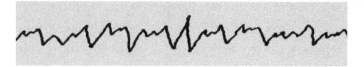

The brain during Stage 4 sleep

It is difficult to wake someone up from Stage 4 sleep even with critical words like 'Fire!' or loud noises such as crashes and crying. When people do wake from Stage 4 sleep, they report no dreams and little or no memory of any ongoing thoughts.

Stage 5 sleep: REM sleep

Finally, we enter rapid eye movement sleep, or dream sleep. During this stage, an EEG reading shows irregular, low-amplitude, fast waves that indicate increased brain activity. But at the same time, our sleep is light. This is why the REM stage is sometimes called 'paradoxical sleep'.

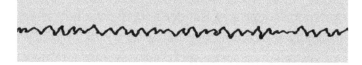

The brain during REM sleep

REM sleep is mostly composed of **beta waves** and other activity that's similar to that of an alert, awake brain. As the name 'REM' suggests, during this stage we can experience variable eye movements and twitches. On the EEG there is little difference from Stage 1 sleep, but if you watch the eye movements of someone experiencing REM sleep, the difference will be clear.

During REM sleep our muscles are more relaxed than in other stages. This particularly applies to the muscles that support our head, which is why we experience a deeper sleep during this stage. Our blood pressure, breathing and heart rate are far more variable than in any of the other stages.

The REM phase of sleep restores our mind, supports memory and learning, and helps our brain clear out irrelevant information: all those important activities we learned about in **Part 1**. It is often assumed that this is when we do *all* our dreaming, but that is not entirely true, as dreams can also occur before and after the REM phase. Up to 90 per cent of dreams that are reported occur when people are awakened during the REM stage, but people can also remember dreams when they are awakened from non-REM stages. During REM sleep, however, we are more likely to have vivid dreams with detailed plots.

REM sleep is closely associated with our biological clock, because even if we go to sleep later, this stage occurs around the same clock time every night. This means our amount of REM does not depend on how long we have been asleep.

Let's look a little more closely at what occurs in the brain during REM sleep. Activity increases particularly in the **pons** and the **limbic system**, both of which are closely linked with our emotional controls. (We'll learn a little more about the limbic system when we look at **EMOTIONS AND STRESS** [pages 55 to 59].)

It is the pons that triggers the REM sleep stage, by releasing a distinctive pattern of high-amplitude electrical waves called **PGO waves**. Soon after they are detected in the pons, they appear in the **lateral geniculate nucleus** of the thalamus, and finally they emerge in the **occipital cortex** – hence the name PGO (pons–geniculate–occipital) waves.

Cells in the pons contribute to REM sleep by sending messages to the **spinal cord** to disable the motor cortex, which controls our body's movements. This means that during REM, our body is paralysed except for occasional twitches, so we are protected from physically acting out our dreams. (We saw in **Part 1** [page 26] that a malfunctioning of this paralysis mechanism may be connected with **sleepwalking**.)

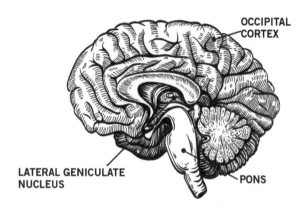

The areas of the brain where PGO waves can be detected

Our 'sleep structure'

There are big differences in the length of sleep cycles and the amount of REM and deep non-REM sleep children and adults of various ages seem to require. The sleep cycle length – the time between two appearances of the same sleep state – increases from about **fifty minutes** in a full-term baby to the adult level of **ninety minutes** by adolescence. (We'll learn a lot more about the sleep cycles of babies, children and adolescents in **Part 4**.)

As adults, our sleep structure is ideally composed of **four to six ninety-minute cycles**. It takes about **eight hours** to get through those four to six cycles.

When we fall asleep, Stage 1 is initiated and lasts about **five minutes**. Then we will normally progress through Stages 2 and 3 in about ten minutes to enter Stage 4, assuming we are not disturbed by any bright light, loud noise or other event. About an hour into our sleep, we begin to cycle back from Stage 4 through Stages 3 and 2 and then REM (Stage 5).

The second cycle ends in the same way as the first. We spend most of the first few hours of the night in **deep, non-dreaming (Stage 4 non-REM) sleep** and the rest of the night alternating between **lighter non-REM (Stage 2) sleep** and

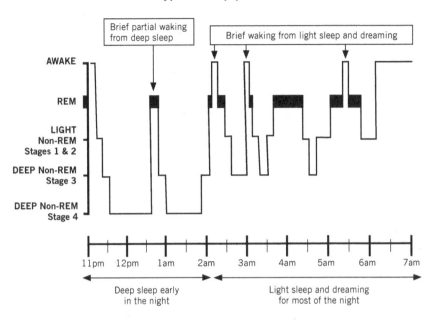

Typical sleep pattern for adults

dreaming **(REM)**. Young children will descend into Stage 3 or 4 before the final waking in the morning, while this is less common in adolescents and adults.

The amount of time we spend in **deep sleep** varies greatly according to age. For young people, this important restorative phase lasts for thirty-minute stretches and accounts for approximately **20 per cent** of total sleep. Unfortunately, after the age of sixty-five, the amount of deep sleep greatly declines, and it may account for no more than **twenty minutes a night** after the age of seventy-five.

REM also accounts for about 20 per cent of our sleep. The dream segments of REM sleep occur about three to five times a night, or about every ninety minutes. Our first REM episode tends to be relatively short, lasting up to ten minutes, and not very intense. There will not be many eye movements, and our breathing and heart patterns will remain fairly stable. As we approach morning, our periods in REM get longer; the final period may last half an hour. The REM periods that appear towards morning are also more intense, with more interesting dreams that can occasionally be scary or even nightmarish.

As our brain moves through the five stages of sleep, it's processing old information and getting itself ready to deal with the challenges that the next day holds. Our goal should be to get as much REM sleep and deep non-REM sleep as possible, to allow for maximum alertness, concentration, creativity and energy, optimal health and a positive mood.

Waking during the night

We all have brief wakings throughout the night, especially during the transitions between non-REM and REM sleep. These short arousals have several functions: we need to change positions for the health of our skin surfaces, muscles and joints; and we need to check for potential dangers, by making sure our surroundings are still the same as they were when we went to sleep. Typically we turn over, straighten the covers and get our pillow back into a preferred position.

These arousals should last only a few seconds or minutes. Assuming all is well, we return to sleep quickly, usually without any memory that the awakening has even occurred. If there are strange noises, however, or other sensory changes (lights, smells etc), we are likely to wake up and explore what is going on. If anything doesn't seem right, we can become more fully alert.

This wakefulness can be a problem for children and, as we'll learn in **Part 4**, it's often based on what they associate with falling asleep. But night-time wakefulness can also happen to adults, for all sorts of reasons. We may suffer from one of the health problems or sleep disorders covered in **Part 1** that interfere with our sleep. We may get up to go to the bathroom, to tell off a noisy neighbour, or to comfort a crying child. Or, as we're about to find out, we may have an issue with our **biological clock**, our body temperature, or our **emotions and stress**.

Waking up and not being able to return to sleep may be just an occasional issue. But if it persists, it can start to rewire our brain or form new habits, so we worry more and more about the problems that are causing our lack of sleep, which then means we get *even less* sleep. Before we know it, this vicious cycle has turned into chronic insomnia.

Getting the basics right

To avoid night-time waking, a good start is to develop some basic healthy habits around sleep. Rule number one: learn to associate your bed only with sleep and 'cuddling' with your partner. If you can't get to sleep, or you wake at night, you may learn to associate bed with lying awake thinking and worrying – so instead, get up after fifteen minutes, go into another room and do something relaxing. It also helps to create a sleep-inducing environment, in which you're less likely to be woken by things like loud noise or a full bladder. You'll find more helpful tips on this in **Part 3**.

But to get a good, even *excellent*, night's sleep, we'll also need to pay attention to our **biological clock**, our **body temperature** and our **emotions and stress**.

OUR BIOLOGICAL CLOCK

Our lives are made up of many rhythms, which include patterns of sleeping and waking, activity and rest, hunger and eating, and fluctuations in body temperature and hormone release. It is important for these cycles to be in harmony if we are to have a sense of wellbeing each day.

Our ability to fall asleep and to stay asleep is closely tied to the timing of these cycles. Typically we fall asleep as our **body temperature** is falling towards a daily minimum, and we wake up as it starts rising to its peak. (We'll look more at body temperature later in **Part 2**.) Our levels of the hormone **cortisol**, secreted by the **adrenal gland**, also drop off early in the night, then progressively rise before we wake up in the morning. If we have to wake up when our temperature and our cortisol levels are still low, we will do so only with great difficulty. Similarly, we may have trouble falling asleep when our body temperature is at its peak.

The natural length of our body's cycles is actually **slightly more than twenty-four hours**; it's closer to twenty-five hours. This is our daily biological clock, or **circadian rhythm**. It's very resistant to interference, and remains steady in the face of oxygen deprivation, many forms of brain damage, alcohol and tranquillisers. (Watches and clocks were of course developed before we fully understood our body cycles, hence the time difference.)

To reset our biological clock each day we need some kind of stimulus. This stimulus is called a **zeitgeber** or 'time-giver', and our most significant zeitgeber is light. Daily rhythms can only become established and maintained in a regular twenty-four-hour pattern if they are set each day by events that always occur at the same times, and the most important of these are waking up in the morning and going to sleep at night. Other cues include noise, temperature, activity and eating needs, but they are not important on their own and tend to supplement the effect of light on our circadian rhythm. If we don't use these signals to guide us, our cycles will run freely at their natural rate and we will operate on a twenty-five-hour day. This means our natural tendency is to stay up a little later each night and get up a little later each morning, both of which are easier for us to do than going to sleep or waking up *earlier*.

Many of us follow this tendency on weekends. We abandon our weekday schedule and expose ourselves to activity, lights and noises at night while also getting up late the following morning. On Monday, when we wake at our normal time for work or school, the biological clock inside us says it is much earlier, and we have difficulty readjusting to our regular schedule.

Our best efforts to influence our sleep cycles by adjusting our clocks are still influenced significantly by the movement of the sun. The best example of this, of course, is when we implement daylight savings and move our clocks forward by one hour. We force ourselves to go to bed at our 'usual bedtime', only it is really an hour earlier. The next morning, when we get up, our brain registers that it's still an hour earlier and we'll feel sluggish for several days before our brains and bodies fully adjust. If we already operate on less sleep, the movement to daylight savings is particularly onerous.

Our sleep is sensitive to *any* light, including artificial light, and our sleep patterns have changed hugely in the past century or so with the introduction of artificial light and heating. Our brain can become quite confused as it seeks darkness and the lowest body temperature for sleep.

With light so important in the resetting of our biological clock, the question you may now be asking is: 'What about blind people?' Like the rest of us, they rely on the secondary zeitgebers of noise, temperature, hunger and activity. To supplement these, blind people have what are called free-running circadian rhythms – as we're about to find out, our brain doesn't need to receive light through our eyes for our circadian rhythm to go on functioning.

The SCN

The part of the brain our biological clock depends on is the **hypothalamus**, and in particular a region called the **suprachiasmatic nucleus** (SCN). We can find the SCN just above the **optic chiasm**, the place where the optic nerves from both our eyes cross, enabling us to see. The SCN is in charge of our circadian rhythms, sleep and body temperature.

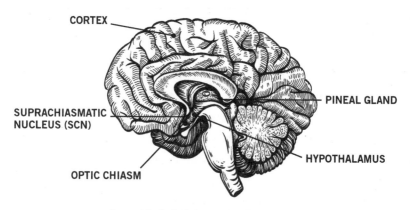

Areas of the brain that control our biological clock

One branch of the optic nerves is called the **retinohypothalamic path**, leading from the **retinas** in the eyes to the SCN. Along the retinohypothalamic path there is a special population of **retinal ganglion cells** that respond directly to light, even if they do not receive input from the retinas' usual light-detecting cells (known as rods and cones). The light they do receive from the eyes supplements their own direct response to light.

These cells respond slowly when light turns on, and turn off slowly when light ceases. Importantly, they respond to the *overall average amount* of light, not to sudden changes. This average intensity over time is the information the SCN needs to calculate what time of day it is.

Research has shown that if SCN neurons are disconnected from the rest of the brain, they continue to produce circadian rhythms, so they are very resilient indeed.

The SCN controls sleep and wakefulness across different parts of the brain, including the **pineal gland**. The role of this gland is to release a hormone known as **melatonin** at night to make us feel sleepy. The retinas in our eyes detect light and send signals to the pineal gland. As the day becomes brighter, the pineal gland produces less melatonin; then, as the daylight fades and night descends, melatonin production increases, promoting sleep.

Our rhythms are innate, not learned, and are genetically controlled. There are **two genes** that produce our circadian rhythm, called **Period** and **Timeless**. They generate proteins in small amounts in the morning, and in increasing amounts as the day progresses. By night time, the Period and Timeless proteins have reached a high level, and combine with another protein called **Clock** to produce sleep. Throughout the night, Period and Timeless no longer produce protein, and the concentration in our body diminishes until the process starts up again in the morning.

The firing of neurons in the brain in response to external light can activate the Timeless protein, which will reduce our sleep and lead to a reset of our biological clock. The key here is that light alters the production of the Period and Timeless proteins and affects the activity of specific neurons in the SCN. An awareness of this helps us to understand a lot about sleep and sleep problems.

Problems with our biological clock

Because our natural rhythms run for slightly longer than twenty-four hours, it's difficult for us to keep to a twenty-four-hour schedule. Brain science began to understand the treatment of sleep disorders when sleep and waking were seen as a rhythm that acts in unison with other body rhythms such as temperature, eating and hormone release.

If we are to achieve better, even *excellent*, sleep, and function at our best during the day, then we need to ensure that these biological rhythms are in sync. Problems occur when our routines are irregular, or when we try to sleep at times that do not match our natural sleep–wake rhythms.

The good news, though, is that problems related to our circadian rhythm are easily correctable. This is the case for most of the people who fall into the categories we're going to look at next.

Sleep phases: larks and owls

When our bedtime and wake-up times do not match our natural sleep–wake rhythms, we will have trouble going to sleep at night and difficulty getting up in the morning, or we will have problems staying awake until bedtime and then wake too early in the morning. When either of these things happens, it means the sleep phase of our sleep–wake cycle is not ideal and needs to be adjusted. It may be too early (**early sleep phase**) or too late (**late sleep phase**).

If we are **sleep-phase-delayed** (have a late sleep phase), we can have trouble falling asleep at the usual time because the hypothalamus (responsible for our circadian rhythm) thinks it is not late enough. We would normally fall asleep while our body temperature is falling, but this fall has not started when we are phase-delayed. On the other hand, someone who is **sleep-phase-advanced** (has an early sleep phase) can fall asleep without any problems but will find themselves waking early as their temperature prematurely begins to rise. An early sleep phase is less common than a late sleep phase, because of our natural tendency to shift later in our twenty-five hour cycle, as previously discussed.

'**Larks**' wake up early full of energy and run out of steam in the evening. (As we'll see in **Part 4**, this is a particular problem for children.) Larks are less likely to let their sleep phase shift late even when they can – on weekends and holidays, for example.

'**Owls**' like to stay up late and wake up late. At any opportunity they are happy to let their sleep–wake schedules move later and later. They feel energetic at night, but do have

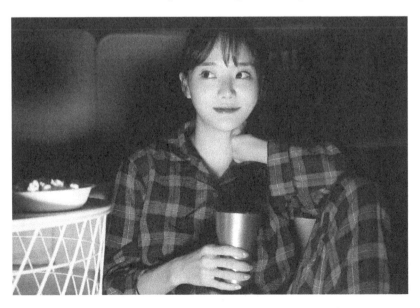

difficulty when they have to wake up in the morning for school or work, regardless of the amount of sleep they've had. They learn to tolerate sleep deprivation reasonably well, and their brain arousal levels, as measured using fMRI (functional magnetic resonance imaging), are often greater than those of the average population.

In fact, we all sleep best if we keep to a regular schedule. Studies have shown that irregular sleep patterns lead to significant alterations in our mood and in our sense of wellbeing, and undermine our ability to sleep at desired times.

We need to be firm with ourselves when it comes to our sleeping and waking times. Learning new routines can be difficult, because our brain looks for repetition to create habits that will minimise energy consumption. The brain will try to stick to the routines we already have in place, but with perseverance and repetition we can start to form more suitable habits.

Shift workers

Shift workers live in a world of very irregular sleep patterns. They must try to sleep when they feel awake and try to get up

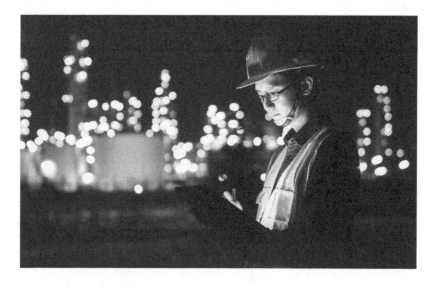

when they feel tired. When their shift requires them to sleep in the morning or early afternoon, and they have been awake for a long time, they still find that they can only sleep briefly. If they change shifts too frequently, their sleep rhythms cannot stabilise and they suffer ongoing sleep problems.

Even after many years of shift work, night-shift workers (midnight to 8am) find that they never adjust completely. They feel sleepy at work because their body temperature continues to peak when they are trying to sleep during the day and not during the night while they are working. Artificial lighting is only partially effective in its ability to reset our body clock. Night-shift workers can only adjust properly if they try to sleep during the day in a very dark room, and use a light at night that is the equivalent of bright daytime light (which is usually between 60 and 400 times brighter than typical levels of artificial lighting in a house).

Jet lag

When we cross time zones and disrupt our biological clock, we often find ourselves feeling sleepy during the day and sleepless at night, with diminished focus and concentration. Some of us we can even feel depressed. The different daylight schedules we experience confuse our brain into thinking it is night time when it's actually daytime. It's very hard for us to catch up on sleep because it's difficult to fall asleep at unexpected times. It usually requires a few days of the new light schedule for our rhythms to reset themselves.

For most of us, travelling across time zones is easier when going from west to east, because we stay awake and get up later, allowing us to partially adjust to the new time zone. Going the other way means we tend to go to sleep earlier, which is before our body's usual bedtime. We've already seen that it's easier for us to sleep in and stay up late than go to bed or wake up early.

Being human means that each of us reacts to time-zone changes differently. When we experience jet lag for longer periods, the neurons located in the hippocampus – our memory storage area – may even be damaged, leading to partial memory loss. This is a particular problem for those who repeatedly have to adjust their time clocks, such as pilots and flight attendants.

Melatonin can be very helpful for those with jet lag, and others who need to sleep at odd hours. Our melatonin levels start to shift upwards about three hours before we go to bed. This means that taking melatonin pills just before bed will have very little effect. A small to moderate dose in the afternoon, however, will advance our biological clock so that we get sleepier in the evening and wake up earlier in the morning.

Melatonin is a popular drug for those experiencing sleep problems, but its long-term effects on humans are unknown. As with any drug, it is best used only when we really need it.

Getting the basics right

All of us need to pay attention to the rhythms of our biological clock – even if we're not a lark or an owl, a shift worker, or someone who changes time zones regularly. We can start by restricting naps during the day. We can avoid light in the bedroom that might keep us awake at night, and we can treat ourselves to lots of it when it's time to wake up.
Part 3 includes more basic tips.

OUR BODY TEMPERATURE

Homeostasis and allostasis

The human body temperature fluctuates from a low of **36.7° Celsius** during the night while we sleep to **37.2° Celsius** in the late afternoon. The brain's regulation of these temperatures is one of the most important functions it has.

On average we use up 2600 kilocalories of energy per day: 30 per cent for all our physical and mental functions, and the other 70 per cent to maintain a constant body temperature, or basal metabolic rate. The key with temperature regulation, as with all other body processes (including sleep), is for the body to keep variables within a fixed range, so it has enough energy left to carry out the other functions that are necessary to keep us alive. This regulation is achieved through the processes of homeostasis and allostasis.

Think of the automatic cruise control in your car. You set a speed and your car maintains that speed in all conditions, by accelerating when going uphill and braking when going downhill – automatically. In just the same manner, **homeostasis** triggers physical and mental activities that automatically maintain certain variables within a set range – for instance, a body temperature of 36.7°C to 37.2°C during daytime.

But when the driving conditions change – for example, you come off the freeway into an urban area – you have to turn off the cruise control and lower your speed. In a similar way, as we head into night the hypothalamus reduces energy usage to a minimum by lowering our body temperature to a fairly constant 36.7°C. We refer to this kind of adaptation to changing conditions as **allostasis**.

Once our body has reached this lower temperature, the process of homeostasis will ensure that it maintains this new set point. Just as a car needs to brake to slow down, we will be awoken to help bring down the temperature if our bedroom becomes too hot. And if we wake fully so that we can make the room cooler, it may have a negative effect on our night's sleep.

Getting the basics right

Apart from keeping our bedroom cool, the best way to avoid heating up too much at night is to stop eating three to five hours before bed. Forcing our body to digest food will heat us up at the time of night when we're meant to be cooling down. On the other hand, a nice warm bath or shower in the hours before bed will mean our body actually cools down by the time we go to sleep. We'll learn more handy tips on body temperature in **Part 3**.

EMOTIONS
AND STRESS

A bedroom that is too hot or cold is one thing, but what about when we can't stop thinking, or are feeling emotional or stressed? How do our homeostatic and allostatic systems regulate our body's operation when our sleep is poor or we can't sleep at all?

Our emotions are essential to the healthy functioning of our brain and body during sleep. The area of the brain responsible for emotional regulation is our **cortex**, and in particular the brain's **limbic system** – the areas of our forebrain surrounding the **thalamus** and the **amygdala**.

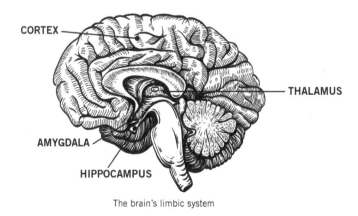

The brain's limbic system

We saw in **Part 1** (page 11) that the amygdala acts as a storage area for memories that arouse emotions, and seems to have an important role in our dreams. Another important part of the limbic system, the **hippocampus**, stores the information we capture with our senses, and helps us associate memories with certain senses (a particular smell etc).

The parasympathetic and sympathetic nervous systems

A key role of our emotions is to protect us from threat. So part of the amygdala's job is to form new memories related to **fear**, helping us to learn which dangers to avoid. A similar function is performed by our sympathetic and **parasympathetic nervous systems**. Just as **homeostasis** keeps our body temperature within a normal range and **allostasis** helps it adapt to external changes, the **parasympathetic nervous system** is responsible for keeping our internal systems running efficiently, while the **sympathetic nervous system** sets off numerous changes within our body in response to possible threat. These include a faster pulse, deeper breathing, a higher blood sugar level and release of the stress hormone adrenaline. But there are many others, as you can see on the **right-hand side** of the diagram opposite.

The sympathetic nervous system is activated by our emotional responses. The purpose of certain emotions is quite clear. When we experience *fear*, we are being alerted to the need to escape from danger. Anger prepares us to fight off an intruder, while *disgust* helps us to avoid things that could make us ill. It generally takes us a micro-second for us to evaluate a situation as dangerous, safe, bad, good etc. But there are many emotions such as embarrassment, sadness and even happiness that are not so obvious in terms of their value to our continued survival.

Our emotions most likely evolved as an adaptive mechanism for our early ancestors. If you've read my previous

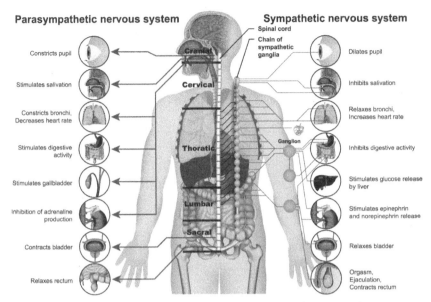

The reactions triggered by our parasympathetic and sympathetic nervous systems

book *The Neuroscience of Mindfulness*, you may remember Brog, our imagined prehistoric forebear from 150,000 years ago. Brog's life was all about survival, which included hunting for food each day. Physical danger was everywhere. If Brog came across a lion, for instance, his body would flood with fear, activating his sympathetic nervous system, and he would have a split second to assess whether to run or stay. We call this the **fight-or-flight** response. Once the threat was over – either because Brog chose to run or because he stayed and won the fight – Brog's parasympathetic nervous system took over and returned his body to its normal calm state. All the activities listed on the *left-hand side* of the diagram above would resume.

Our world today is very different from Brog's. We buy our food at the supermarket, and the only lions we encounter are safely behind bars at the zoo. But even though our lives are so much more sophisticated than Brog's, our bodies still work in exactly the same way. The big problem is that *real, external* threats have been largely replaced by *internal anxieties* over situations we only *perceive* as threatening or stressful.

Major events – divorce, death of a loved one, moving house, changing jobs – can upend our lives for some time. But other stresses are constant. Modern technology means we're perpetually surrounded by stressful events via our phones, laptops and other devices. It also means we're expected to do twice as much, in half the time. We're in the middle of a stress pandemic. And even though our conscious mind tells us that these emotional threats aren't the same as being confronted by a hungry lion, our *unconscious* mind can't tell the difference. Our fight-or-flight response is permanently activated. Our brains are swirling with constant activity, racing from one thing to the next all day long. We find it difficult to 'turn off'. Our bodies simply weren't designed to cope with this kind of chronic stress.

The mind–body connection

The Greek philosopher Galen talked about the mind–body connection way back in the second century. In the early twentieth century the Harvard physiology professor Walter Cannon published a paper demonstrating the relationship between emotions and digestion. Later, in the 1930s, endocrinologist Hans Selye became the first to describe the modern concept of stress while studying physiological responses to, well, what everyone now calls stress.

When Selye was doing research on dogs, he found very specific changes in their bodies due to emotions such as anger, fear and anxiety. When their bodies were under continual stress he found changes such as ulcers, swelling of the adrenal cortex (in the adrenal glands, which rest above the kidneys) and deterioration of the thymus gland (in the centre of the upper chest). This research was later applied to the human body. It showed that changes in living and working situations could positively or negatively affect our health in noticeable ways. (You can read a lot more about the mind–body connection in my book *The Neuroscience of Mindfulness*.)

These stresses have even greater impacts on our health when they spill over into our sleep. Most of us have nights when we're unable to stop thinking about events, even when we're sure we're not thinking about them. Unfortunately our subconscious systems don't play along with our conscious thoughts, and continue to process the emotions associated with those events. If the events are threatening or negative, and linked to overwhelming stress, they may infringe on our sleep.

We learned earlier that brief partial awakenings during the night are perfectly normal, particularly when transitioning between REM and non-REM sleep. But if our brains are still consumed by the events of our day, we'll wake fully and we'll stay awake. This may develop into chronic insomnia.

Daytime events can have other long-term sleep impacts too. If we can't stop worrying about negative events, our memories of them may be filed inappropriately by our brain's cortex. If this happens, our brain will not be able to routinely sift through and process the information properly, and we'll have no control over how or when the events will resurface.

Getting the basics right

There are so many basic things we can do to avoid letting stress and worry affect our sleep. We can avoid thinking about things that will upset us before bed, or doing things that will get our brain and body too excited. We can start to establish habits and rituals that will tell our body it's time for bed. Or we can do any of the exercises we're about to look at in **Part 3**, which are all specifically designed to combat the effects of stress and leave us relaxed before bedtime.

But to get to get to the root of the problem, we'll need to work at eliminating those negative emotions and stresses from our life altogether. (This is one of main topics of *The Neuroscience of Mindfulness*; it may be the *next* book you need to read.)

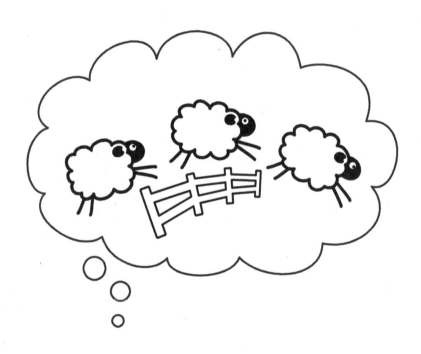

PART 3

HOW TO GET AN
EXCELLENT SLEEP

'The worst thing in the world is to try
to sleep and not to.'

—F. Scott Fitzgerald, American author (1896–1940)

At some point in our lives we all wish we could get to sleep quicker, and sleep longer, deeper or simply with fewer interruptions. This is part of the journey towards achieving *excellent sleep*. Let's start by working out how good our current sleep is, then learn to master the basics of a good night's sleep. Once we've got them covered, we'll be ready to prepare our brain and body for *excellent sleep* with exercises we can do either during the day, or before or after sleep.

They're going to take some effort, but if we really want to improve and not just stay where we are, then the effort will be truly worthwhile.

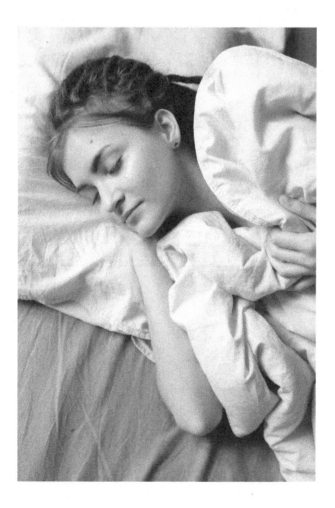

EXCELLENT SLEEP QUIZ

To achieve *excellent sleep*, we first need to understand our current level of sleep. Complete the sleep quiz that follows to see just how good your sleep is at the moment. By improving in the areas where you're currently not doing so well, you will be on your way to achieving *excellent sleep*.

A. Sleep duration and quality

1. How much sleep did you get last night?

____hours____minutes

2. What was the quality of your sleep – how did you feel when you woke up?

__ /10 where 10 = good

3. How long did you take to fall asleep?

___hours___minutes

4. If you woke up during the night, how long were you awake?

____hours___minutes

B. Sleep patterns

Do you tend to …

5. Have trouble falling asleep?

YES/NO

6. Have trouble falling asleep *and* waking up?
YES/NO

7. Fall asleep OK but wake up early or in the middle of the night?
YES/NO

8. Have no fixed bedtime?
YES/NO

9. Think you spend too much time in bed?
YES/NO

10. Go to bed and get up at times that allow you to get eight hours' sleep?
YES/NO

C. The hours before bed

Do you ...

11. Drink coffee in the late afternoon or early evening?
YES/NO

12. Drink alcohol after dinner?
YES/NO

13. Smoke cigarettes before bed?
YES/NO

14. Eat sugary, fatty or high-protein foods before bed?
YES/NO

15. Eat within three to five hours of going to bed?
YES/NO

16. Have a warm bath for ten to twenty minutes in the hours before bed?
YES/NO

D. Just before sleep

Do you ...

17. Practise a bedtime ritual (e.g. reading a book) to let your body know it is time to sleep?
YES/NO

18. Go to bed at your usual time even if you aren't sleepy?
YES/NO

19. Have a clock that you can see when you're in bed?
YES/NO

20. Watch TV or use your laptop, tablet or mobile phone before sleep?
YES/NO

21. Think or talk about the things you have to do tomorrow before going to sleep?
YES/NO

E. Trouble sleeping

Do you ...

22. Get up, go into another room and do something relaxing if you are not asleep within about fifteen minutes?
YES/NO

23. Get up during the night and eat, drink or have a cigarette?
YES/NO

24. Lie in bed and worry if you can't sleep?
YES/NO

F. During the day

Do you ...

25. Have a fixed time to get up?
YES/NO

26. Open your blinds or curtains or turn on the light when you get up?
YES/NO

27. Have a nap of more than thirty minutes during the day?
YES/NO

28. Avoid lying down during the day except when you are trying to sleep?
YES/NO

29. Practise any relaxation techniques during the day?
YES/NO

30. Often feel worried and anxious and/or sad and miserable during the day?
YES/NO

Scoring

A (questions 1 to 4): this information about your sleeping is only to enhance your awareness of your current sleep patterns.

B to F (questions 5 to 30): give yourself one point for each of the following responses.

Q 5	NO	Q 14	NO	Q 23	NO
Q 6	NO	Q 15	NO	Q 24	NO
Q 7	NO	Q 16	YES	Q 25	YES
Q 8	NO	Q 17	YES	Q 26	YES
Q 9	NO	Q 18	NO	Q 27	NO
Q 10	YES	Q 19	NO	Q 28	YES
Q 11	NO	Q 20	NO	Q 29	YES
Q 12	NO	Q 21	NO	Q 30	NO
Q 13	NO	Q 22	YES		

0–5 **Very poor**
6–10 **Poor**
11–16 **Average**
17–22 **Good**
23–26 **Excellent**

Not sure how to improve your bad score? Start by **getting the basics right**. Read on to find out how ...

GETTING THE BASICS RIGHT

In **Part 2**, we learned about what happens when we sleep, and about some of the things that can stop us from getting an *excellent sleep*. We learned that we need to create a sleep-inducing environment so we're less likely to wake when transitioning from one sleep stage to another. We learned that we need to follow our biological clock, to keep our body temperature low, and to relax our brain and body to avoid being woken by negative emotions and stress.

As with anything in life, the key to achieving the best possible sleep is proper preparation. And that starts with getting the basics right. As we'll see from the tips below, preparing for an *excellent sleep* starts as early as when we first wake up in the morning.

Creating a sleep-inducing environment

- ✍ **Learn to associate your bed only with sleeping and 'cuddling'.** Don't eat, watch TV or gather the family to hang out in bed.

- ✍ For the same reason, if you are not asleep within about **fifteen minutes** – or wake up later and stay awake for around that time – **get up, go into another room and do something relaxing** until you feel sleepy again.

@ **Don't watch the clock** once you go to bed. (If you have trouble sleeping you'll have to estimate when those fifteen minutes are up.)

@ To avoid waking up at night with a full bladder, try not to **drink any fluids** in the two hours before bed.

@ Wear **earplugs** if you can hear noises from outside your room.

@ Try a **white-noise maker**, which emits a combination of sounds of different frequencies to mask outside noises and help condition your brain to know when it's time to sleep. Choose a brand that makes different sounds, so you can choose the one/s that work/s best for you.

@ Use a **humidifier** if you feel congested or the air is especially dry.

Following your biological clock

@ To avoid disturbing your circadian rhythm, avoid **lying down during the day** except when trying to **nap**. Make sure you nap for no longer than thirty minutes, and before 3pm.

@ Maintain a regular bedtime schedule. Go to bed and wake up at the same time every day, including weekends, even if it occasionally means losing sleep. Try to get **eight hours' sleep** a night.

@ Sleep in **complete darkness**. If necessary, use blackout drapes to keep out light from outside. Light is the main stimulus that resets your biological clock each day, so too much of it during the night will make your body think it's time to wake up.

- Wear **eyeshades** to cover your eyes if you want things even darker.

- Avoid alarm clocks or other electronic devices with **lighted displays** that you can see from bed.

- Avoid using **loud alarm clocks**. Consider one that gently turns on the radio or makes noises that gradually grow louder. To wake up properly, **your brain needs to clearly differentiate between being asleep and being awake**. Suddenly being woken out of deep sleep by a loud alarm leaves you half-asleep as you begin your day.

- Expose yourself to **bright light** as soon as you get up by turning on a light and/or opening your blinds or curtains. Even better, go outside and take some deep breaths of **fresh air**, or do some **exercise**. These activities will wake up your brain and body in a healthy way.

- Better still, do any of the **brain exercises** on pages 85 to 124 that are designed to be used when you wake up.

Keeping your body temperature low

- Keep your bedroom **cool and well ventilated**. Turn down the thermostat two hours before bedtime.

- Try to **avoid eating** within **three to five hours** of going to bed. Otherwise, your digestive system will need to start working, raising your body temperature just when it's meant to be cooling down. However, don't go to bed hungry, which will also make it hard to get to sleep.

- Avoid **sugary** foods, which will force your pancreas to start producing insulin and raise your blood sugar level, keeping you awake.

- At your last meal of the day, avoid **foods that are high in protein**, which take a long time to break down, make your stomach release acid, and may give you heartburn.

- Avoid **fatty** foods for the same reasons; they take even longer to break down in the stomach.

- Avoid other foods that give you **heartburn**, such as spicy foods, peppermint and onions.

- Avoid **caffeinated** foods and drinks – chocolate, coffee, tea and soft drinks – as the caffeine will keep you awake.

- Avoid **alcohol**, which will force your liver to start digesting it.

- Avoid **smoking**, as nicotine is a stimulant that will keep you awake. Of course, it's best to quit entirely.

- Avoid **getting up during the night to eat, drink or smoke**. This will have all the same effects as doing those things three to five hours before bed, and will guarantee that you'll have difficulty getting back to sleep.

- Try to have a **hot bath** for ten to twenty minutes an hour and a half before bed. As well as increasing your circulation, the heat radiated by your body will actually cool you down by bedtime.

Relaxing your brain and body for sleep

- Do any of the **brain exercises** in Part 4 that are designed to be used during the day.

- Vigorous **exercise** during the day is great to release pent-up stress, but avoid exercising for two to four hours before bedtime.

- Avoid **'busy work'** for two hours before bed, including house-cleaning and paying bills.

- Avoid playing **stimulating computer games** for two hours before bedtime.

- Maintain a **healthy relationship** with your partner, family and friends. Resolve minor disputes before going to bed, but postpone more difficult discussions until everyone involved has had a good night's sleep.

- Avoid **stewing over problems** before bedtime. As we've seen, stress, anxiety and depression are common reasons for insomnia. Instead, work on solutions to your problems during the day.

- Avoid thinking or talking about **the things you need to do the next day** before bed. Some people find that writing them down helps them avoid worrying about these issues during the night.

- Spend the hour before going to bed unwinding and **mentally separating yourself** from the day.

- Signal to yourself that it's time to become sleepy with **bedtime activities** such as brushing your teeth or turning out the lights.

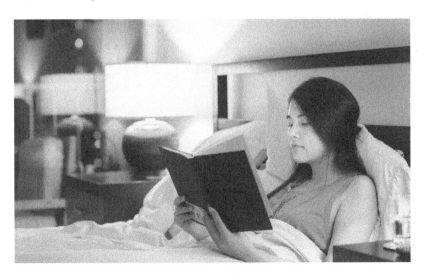

- Establish a **relaxing bedtime ritual**, such as reading a book, or having someone rub your back.

- If you do **read** before bed, avoid anything stimulating, like action or horror novels.

- Avoid **television** before bedtime, and keep the TV out of your bedroom.

- Avoid looking at devices such as **laptops**, **tablets** and **mobile phones** before bed, and keep them out of the bedroom too.

- Do deep, rhythmic **breathing** before sleep. Breathe slowly as if you were already asleep. Or try **relaxation breathing** (page 90).

- Do any of the **brain exercises** on pages 106 to 124 that are designed to be used before sleep.

Being realistic

- Develop more realistic expectations about sleep. It's *not* realistic to assume that you *have* to fall asleep as soon as your head hits the pillow, that you *always* have to get eight hours of uninterrupted sleep, that you should never wake up during the night, or that should *always* feel rested and energised the next day. Aiming for perfection can cause you to develop performance anxiety about sleep, which will probably make your sleep worse.

A MULTI-SENSORY TECHNIQUE FOR EXCELLENT SLEEP

Peppermint tea
(TASTE & SMELL)

Colouring in
(SIGHT)

Binaural beats
technology
(SOUND)

Colouring in
(TOUCH)

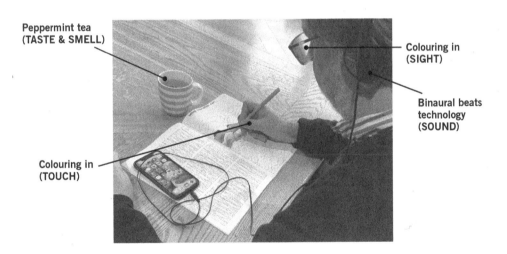

If we want to be *excellent* at anything, we definitely need to practise and prepare – and this includes sleep. During the day we need to ensure that our brain remains as relaxed and stress-free as possible. We're going to learn in this section how to do this by engaging the brain through its only communication channels: **our five senses**.

Sight and touch

Using sight and touch while practising **relaxation breathing** (which we'll learn about on page 90) is a powerful method to help us with acute and chronic stress situations that often lead to poor sleep.

For many of us, however, just the breathing component is challenging. Common responses include:

'I DON'T HAVE TIME.'
'I KEEP FORGETTING TO DO IT.'
'I CAN'T STAY FOCUSED, SO WHY BOTHER?'
'I DON'T KNOW HOW TO DO IT RIGHT.'
'IT DOESN'T WORK FOR ME.'
'I KEEP FALLING ASLEEP.'
'I FEEL SILLY DOING IT, AND IT'S BORING.'

To get over these perceptions, we need to calm our brain both in the short (acute) term and in the long (chronic) term. **Colouring in** is an activity that for most of us is associated with times and places in which we have felt happy and secure. The brain recognises this, and immediately opens neural pathways that it associates with these feelings.

Brain science enhances the calming effect by using drawings specifically developed to have the biggest possible impact on the brain while we colour them in. When we're doing this, we are practising **mindfulness**, which involves *being aware of where we are in the moment, and being able to focus on the activity that we're doing, to the exclusion of everything else.*

We can practise mindfulness in lots of other ways too, even while doing everyday activities such as brushing or combing our hair, or going for a walk. (You'll find a few ideas in my book *The Neuroscience of Mindfulness*.) For now, though, we're going to concentrate on **mindful colouring**.

The drawings we choose should emphasise:

1. Pattern

2. Repetition

3. Control

Our brain loves to create **patterns** from **repetition** and within **boundaries**. That's what it's built for. Our brain relaxes even more when the images allow **creativity** in a **non-competitive** way.

The science behind mindful colouring has been proven in my own research using EEG data. Colouring in was shown to lead to an improved heart rate, and in particular heart-rate variation, which we know results in the production of restful **alpha brain waves**. As we saw in **Part 2** (page 35), these are the waves our brain produces just before it enters Stage 1 of sleep.

The image below shows a subject's heart rate at the top and the pulse wave, or heart-rate variation, at the bottom. Colouring in results in deeper breathing and bigger, wider waves, which indicate that the brain is in a relaxed mode.

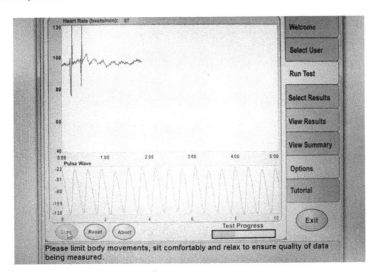

The effect on the brain of mindful colouring

EXERCISE
Mindful colouring

Get yourself an adult colouring-in book. My brain-based colouring books are available at **www.colourtation.com**.

Pick any drawing you like. Choose a colour, focus on the task of colouring and enjoy it for what it is. Also remember:

1. You don't have to finish the whole picture – you can come back to it next time.

2. Let your colour choices just come to you.

3. Be precise and stay within the lines.

4. Let yourself become immersed in the activity and focus on colouring to the exclusion of everything else.

5. Take as little or as much time as you can manage – five minutes should be the minimum.

6. Colour in at least once a day to train your brain to relax, or whenever you feel pressured and stressed.

7. **Make this part of your bedtime routine to prepare your brain to create sleep-inducing alpha waves. This will help you not only go to sleep but also achieve *excellent* sleep.**

Sound

Using sound can make a real difference to our stress and sleep. Most of us already know how easy it is to fall asleep while listening to relaxing music. It really helps us let go of our active thoughts and quieten our mind.

Neuroscience takes this link between sound (music) and behaviour (relaxation and sleep) one step further, by harnessing the brain's responsiveness to sound and transporting us into a state of deeper relaxation, less anxiety and *excellent sleep*.

The fascinating field of soundwave science has led to the development of **binaural beats technology**. In our labs at the MIND Peak Performance Institute, we have tested this exciting technology and seen the dramatic effects on **alpha-wave** production, which helps us turn off our brain, relax and sleep better. For more information, see mindpeakperformance.com/ssplus.

Let's look at this technology more closely. Binaural beats are a technique of combining two slightly different sound frequencies to create the perception of a single new frequency tone. This technology exposes you to two different frequencies at the same time, one in each ear, but the brain actually perceives a single tone that is the difference between the two separate frequencies. When exposed to soundwaves at certain frequencies, brain-wave patterns adjust to align with those frequencies. Your brain, in a sense, tunes itself to the new frequency: a process known as **entrainment**.

You can listen to binaural beats using earphones plugged directly into your mobile phone. In each ear, you receive sound at a slightly different frequency, accompanied by some relaxing background sounds. If your left ear receives a 320-Hz tone and your right ear receives a 310-Hz tone, your brain will process and absorb a 10-Hz tone. That's a very low-frequency soundwave – one you can't actually hear. But you don't need to hear the sound for your brain to be affected by it.

Why is exposure to these soundwaves helpful for sleep and relaxation? Research indicates that it can create changes in the brain's degree of arousal. Listening to sounds that create a low-frequency tone triggers a slowing down of brain-wave activity, which helps us relax, lowers our anxiety, and makes it easier for us to fall asleep and sleep soundly.

But binaural beats don't just help with sleep and relaxation by lowering brain-wave frequency. Some small-scale studies have found that exposure to binaural beats is associated with changes to three hormones important to sleep and wellbeing:

1. **DHEA**. DHEA functions as a kind of master hormone, helping to produce other hormones in the body on an as-needed basis. DHEA is critical to immune function and protection against disease. Particularly significant for sleep is that DHEA works to suppress cortisol (see below). One study found that 68 per cent of participants had increased levels of DHEA after using binaural beats technology.

2. **Cortisol**. As we learned when we looked at **OUR BIOLOGICAL CLOCK** (pages 44 to 52), cortisol is an arousal hormone, stimulating alertness and attention. Cortisol levels rise and fall in connection with circadian rhythms, and are at their peak first thing in the morning, just in time for us to be active for the day. But at elevated levels, cortisol can also provoke stress. Overly high cortisol levels are associated with insomnia, as well as more time spent in light sleep rather than deep sleep. The study referred to above found that 70 per cent of participants experienced a reduction in cortisol after exposure to binaural beats.

3. **Melatonin**. As we also saw on page 47, melatonin promotes and regulates sleep. Melatonin levels rise dramatically in the evening, and the hormone works to relax our body and mind, preparing us to fall asleep. The same study found 73 per cent of participants had higher levels of melatonin after using binaural beats. The average increase was more than 97 per cent.

A growing body of research suggests that, in addition to improving sleep, binaural beats can help mood and mental performance, and reduce different forms of anxiety, from mild to chronic. A couple of especially interesting studies looked at the effects of binaural beats on patients preparing to undergo surgery: a life circumstance that is anxiety-provoking for anyone. They found that binaural beats led to significantly reduced anxiety levels and lower blood-pressure levels.

Using binaural beats technology is an easy shortcut to the meditative state required for *excellent sleep*. An ear-pampering alternative is **alpha sounds**, a soundtrack of sounds in soothing alpha frequencies (see mindpeakperformance.com/ssplus). It lasts just under seven minutes, which is a useful length for a mindful pick-me-up – as you'll see in some of the exercises later.

Smell and taste

Whether it's the delicious aroma of freshly baked banana bread or roasted vegetables, the natural perfume of lavender soap, the scent of flowers in a park or pine trees in a forest, smells can have a powerful effect on our wellbeing, and **aromatherapy** is a proven way to relax the brain and prepare it for sleep. We can help create a sleep-inducing atmosphere with the natural aromas from flowers or essential oils.

Ninety-nine per cent of **taste** is in fact **smell**, so in order to calm your busy mind, try eating and drinking **mindfully**. Take a moment to inhale a piping-hot mug of your favourite tea. Swish it around in your mouth and notice the distinct flavours – are they sweet, sour, bitter, salty or savoury? Slowly and deeply breathe in the scents of your food, appreciating where it came from and how it was made. Notice the distinct flavours and textures, how they pair together, and how different ingredients make you feel.

To prepare yourself for *excellent sleep*, eat and drink at a slower pace, appreciating and savouring every bite and every sip.

A multi-sensory stress management study

At MIND Peak Performance, we believe that to achieve reduced stress and anxiety together with *excellent sleep* we need to use all our senses. To test this we conducted a study to evaluate the effects of our Multi-sensory Stress Management Program. We hoped that it would significantly reduce stress, improve heart-rate variability, decrease blood pressure and improve work performance and sleep.

The study compared ninety-one office workers under stress because their company was downsizing, with seventy-nine healthy control subjects.

The Multi-sensory Stress Management Program took twelve minutes a day – at any time of the day – for thirty days. In those twelve minutes, participants would:

- listen to alpha soundwaves on earphones connected to their phones

- while listening, mindfully colour in a drawing from one of my adult colouring books

- while listening and colouring in, smell and drink a cup of peppermint tea

At the end of the thirty days, those who participated in the Multi-sensory Stress Management Program were significantly less stressed. The other group showed the same scores before and after the sham program.

For the stressed workers, lower stress levels led to improved work performance – and much better sleep. My Multi-sensory Technique for Excellent Sleep could work the same way for you.

THE DECAF
NAPPUCCINO

While working with gamers engaged in elite-level esports over the last few years, I became aware of a technique many of them used to keep themselves refreshed and alert, called the **nappuccino**. The nappuccino worked on the basis that a nap of no more than thirty minutes would refresh the brain. On the downside, the gamers weren't very alert immediately afterwards, so to deal with this they would use caffeine. Caffeine kicks in after twenty minutes, so the technique required them to drink coffee before having a nap of twenty minutes. On awakening, not only would they be refreshed, but their brain would also be stimulated, alert and ready to play.

The problem with this technique is that the medium- to long-term effects of caffeine on the brain are not great. The idea was good, but the components poor. So, to create a healthier version of the technique – a decaf nappuccino, if you like – we rearranged its stages and replaced the coffee with **brain–mind stretching exercises** (see page 85) that would help stimulate the brain immediately after the nap time was completed. These exercises can also be used any time you're having trouble sleeping, or whenever you feel stressed.

Several studies have shown that if you are exposed to information in the morning and tested on it in the late afternoon, you'll perform better if you take a nap (or do some colouring) in between. But remember that you shouldn't force napping – nap if you feel like it, otherwise don't. To repeat what we learned in **GETTING THE BASICS RIGHT** (pages 67 to 72), try to nap before 3pm, and make sure you set a timer so you don't nap longer than thirty minutes. If you do sleep longer you'll start the process towards deep sleep and suffer the effects of a disturbed circadian rhythm.

Waking up the brain

The nappuccino technique raises the question of how long after you start to wake up do you *actually* wake up? Gaining full consciousness can be a very long process. As we learned in **GETTING THE BASICS RIGHT** for *excellent sleep* it is important to clearly define the difference between being asleep and being awake. You can condition your brain to know when it's time to sleep and time to be awake, but if the difference between sleep and wakefulness is left vague, your brain's response when you try to fall asleep or stay asleep will be equally vague. You'll spend long periods being *half asleep* or *half awake*. This is particularly true after you've had a nap.

Never just roll out of bed after sleep, but take the time to **stretch** your body and brain. While the brain has no actual muscles to stretch, it does use chemical and electrical messages to stimulate and relax nerve activity, which is a little like the process of stretching.

If you were going for a run you would stretch your muscles to prepare them. Sudden excessive use of the muscles would probably lead to pain and potential damage. Stretching and increasing the blood flow to your muscles prepares them for heightened use.

When you produce these voluntary body movements you activate a part of the brain called the **(primary) motor cortex**. (As we saw on pages 12 and 40, the motor cortex is shut down during REM sleep to prevent us from moving about during our dreams.) The motor cortex is the width of a headband and runs across the top of the head from one ear to the other. Its function is to control the movements of your body – such as running.

This function was first discovered in 1870 by German scientists Gustav Fritsch and Eduard Hitzig, who conducted experiments on dogs and found that when they stimulated different parts of a dog's motor cortex, different muscles in its body contracted. As the diagram below suggests, fine body movements such as hand and facial movements take up more motor cortex space than larger ones.

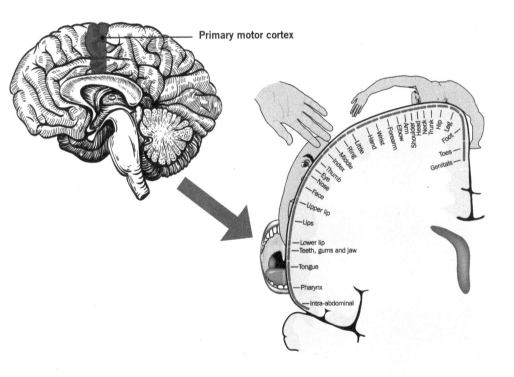

Primary motor cortex

A cross-section of the brain's motor cortex

The exercises on the following pages focus on the **hands** and **fingers**, which means you will be stimulating and relaxing a large area of the motor cortex and affecting as many nearby regions of the cortex as possible. The goal is to activate neurons that will 'stretch' the brain.

Just like physical stretching, brain-stretching involves both 'push' and 'pull'. The motor cortex and surrounding regions of the cortex need to be **stimulated**, then **relaxed**. You'll see that each exercise below involves the use of **breathing**. The physical stimulus of the exercise is counterbalanced by the mental relaxation of the breathing.

Just like physical stretching, these exercises will prepare your brain to go beyond its comfort level, enabling it to respond far better to the mind pressures you experience daily. If you have the tools available, I recommend that you use **mindful colouring in** (pages 92 to 97) and **binaural beats** (page 77) in conjunction with these exercises.

Exercising the hands and fingers stimulates and relaxes the brain, which will help you cope better with mental stress.

EXERCISES
Brain–mind stretching

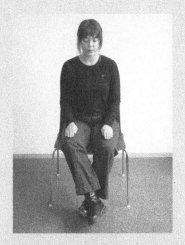

Exercise 1: Sitting on a chair, take a deep breath in through your nose while tensing your leg muscles by crossing your feet at the ankles and pressing down with your upper leg while trying to lift the lower leg. Hold for the count of three, then relax and breathe out through your mouth until your lungs are empty. Repeat three times.

Exercise 2: With your hands in your lap and palm against palm, take a deep breath in through your nose while pressing down with your top hand and trying to lift your lower hand. Hold for the count of three, then relax and breathe out through your mouth until your lungs are empty. Repeat three times.

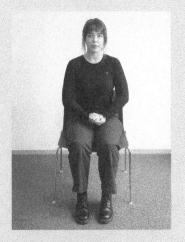

continued

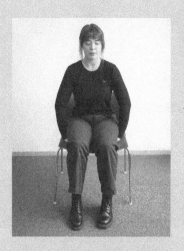

Exercise 3: Place your hands under your thighs and take a deep breath in through your nose while trying to lift your hands up. Hold for the count of three, then relax and breathe out through your mouth until your lungs are empty. Repeat three times.

Exercise 4: Place your hands under the sides of your chair and take a deep breath in through your nose while pulling your hands up. Hold for the count of three, then relax and breathe out through your mouth until your lungs are empty. Repeat three times.

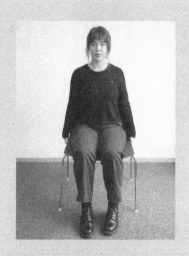

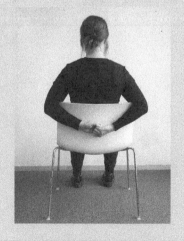

Exercise 5: Grasp your hands behind your chair then take a deep breath in through your nose while trying to pull them apart and simultaneously pushing them in against the back of the chair. Hold for the count of three, then relax and breathe out through your mouth until your lungs are empty. Repeat three times.

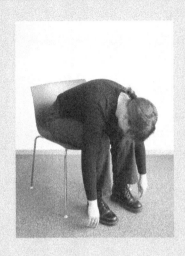

Exercise 6: With both feet flat on the floor, take a deep breath in through your nose and drop your head towards your knees. Let your arms dangle freely. Hold for the count of three, then relax and breathe out through your mouth until your lungs are empty. Repeat three times.

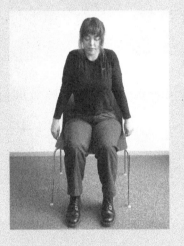

Exercise 7: Take a deep breath in through your nose and shrug your shoulders. Hold for the count of three, then relax and breathe out through your mouth until your lungs are empty. Repeat three times.

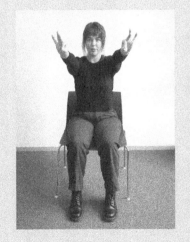

Exercise 8: Take a deep breath in through your nose and extend your arms in front of you, spreading your fingers. Then, one by one, touch the tip of each finger to your thumb. Do this three times while holding your breath, then relax and breathe out through your mouth until your lungs are empty. Repeat three times.

continued

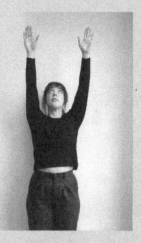

Exercise 9: Stand up. Take a deep breath in through your nose, tilt your head backwards and throw up your arms as if you were trying to touch the roof. Hold for the count of three, then relax and breathe out through your mouth until your lungs are empty. Repeat three times.

These brain–mind stretching exercises can be used any time you feel stressed or anxious or can't sleep. When you combine them with colouring in and binaural beats, you will have a highly effective way of combatting the stressors of daily life.

DAYTIME BRAIN
EXERCISES FOR
EXCELLENT SLEEP

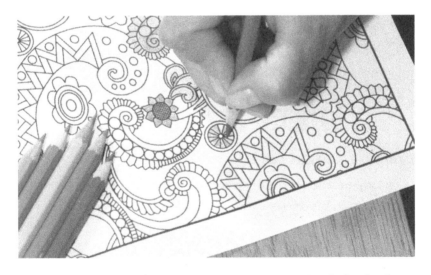

To achieve *excellent sleep*, we need to keep our brain in the best possible condition. As we've seen, during sleep our brain is extremely busy, so the better it functions during the day, the better the results at night. You can use some or all of these exercises *during the day* to improve your brain's performance *both while awake and while asleep.*

Relaxation breathing

EXERCISE
Micro-break breathing

Learn to change your brain from an allostatic (busy) to a homeostatic (balanced) state.

Breathe in through your nose, counting to three: '1 ... 2 ... 3.' Still holding your breath, say the word 'STOP' in your head.

Exhale through your mouth, slowly counting to five: '1 ... 2 ... 3 ... 4 ... 5.'

Make sure you completely empty your lungs while concentrating on a feeling of calm.

Repeat three times.

Micro-breaks must be done at least twice a day to ensure your brain and body remain balanced. Pick a time in the morning and a time in the afternoon.

This exercise can also be used just before high-pressure events that may cause you stress.

Creating a brain edge

Let's look at what typically happens inside our brain as we play a computer game.

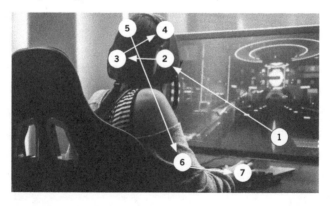

1. Our brain reacts to the movement of an object on the computer screen.

2. Our eyes register the movement and send the information to our two **occipital lobes**, our visual processing centres, located on either side of the back of our skull.

3. The occipital lobes send visual information about the moving object to our **frontal lobes**, our action centres.

4. Our frontal lobes decide that the object on the screen must move left and forward to achieve our goal of winning the game.

5. Our **motor cortex** receives instructions from our frontal lobes, and sends motor control signals to our **spinal cord**.

6. These signals travel along the spinal cord to whichever hand we're using to play the game.

7. That hand moves in specific directions to achieve the goal decided by the frontal lobes.

(**Note:** While the steps above are typical, they are by no means universal. Each of us is unique, and each of our brains is unique too.)

You can see what a complex process our brain goes through to allow our hand to perform even a simple sequence of movements while we're at our computer. Whether we're gaming or using our computer for work, study or fun, we can *create a brain edge* – an improvement in our thinking capability – by doing the following simple exercise.

EXERCISE
20/20/20

Every **20 minutes** you are at a computer screen, look up from the screen, or get up from your desk, and find something **20 metres** away to focus on. Focus on this for **20 seconds** before returning to what you were doing.

Mindful colouring

Here are some variations on the 'Mindful colouring' exercise we looked at on page 76 that you can do during the day to treat your brain and connect with your emotions.

EXERCISE
Brain coding

At your table or desk, at least twice a day, turn away from your computer and colour in the drawing opposite. (Make copies so you can colour it in over and over again.) Start by using the 'Micro-break breathing' you learned in Exercise 1 (page 90).

Continue colouring for at least five minutes. Finishing the picture is *not* required. What is needed is for you to *focus* on the process of colouring. Concentrate on relaxing and feel yourself change from an allostatic (active) state to a *homeostatic* (relaxed) state. The brain loves this.

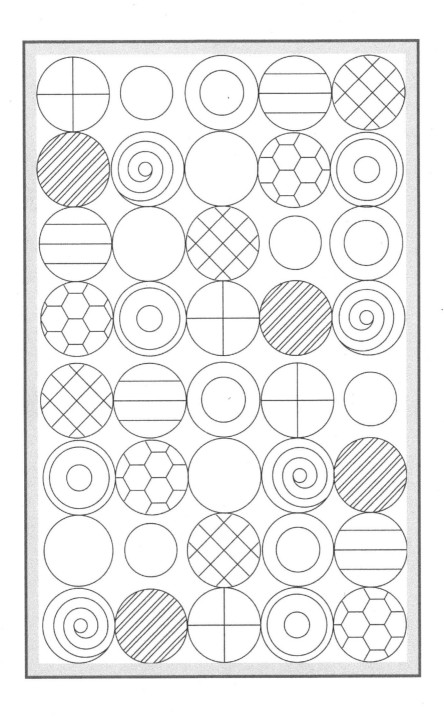

EXERCISE
Emotional DNA

At your table or desk, at least twice a day, turn away from your computer and take out this book (or a copy of the drawing opposite).

Also take out your earphones, attach them to your phone or computer, and listen to the seven-minute alpha soundtrack at mindpeakperformance.com/ssplus.

Before you start colouring and playing the soundtrack, try to picture a colour that will help you stay focused. Use a colour that is significant or pleasing to you. Experiment with different colours until you find the best one(s) for you. Let your colour choices just come to you.

The list below shows some of the emotions I've found are commonly linked to certain colours by people using my *Colourtation* colouring books.

White	Frustrated, confused, bored
Black	Harassed, overworked, tense
Grey	Nervous, strained
Dark blue	Happy, passionate, romantic
Blue	Relaxed, calm, at ease, loving
Pink	Fearful, uncertain, questioning
Purple	Sensual, clear, purposeful
Red	Excited, energised, adventurous, ready to go
Orange	Full of ideas, wanting, daring
Brown	Full of jittery anticipation, restless thoughts
Dark green	Emotion-charged, somewhat relaxed
Mid-green	Average, not under stress, reasonably active
Light green	Unsettled, cool, full of mixed emotions
Yellow	Imaginative, feeling OK, wandering

Now, start colouring. Your intention is to relax for the next seven minutes. Be aware of what you are doing and focus on the pattern you are creating. Use colours that have meaning to you.

When the alpha sounds stop, the exercise is complete. If you want to continue longer, no problem; you just need to keep going for a *minimum of seven minutes*.

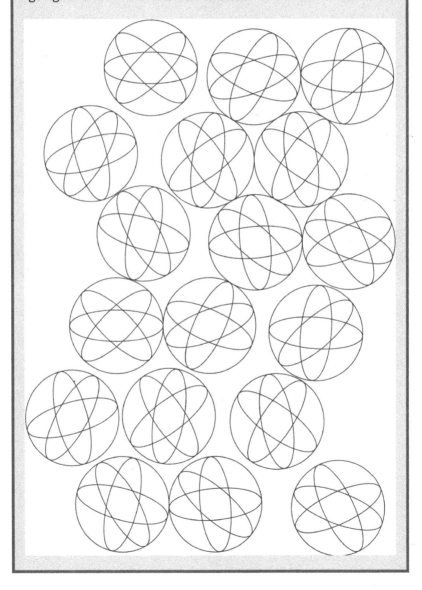

Neuroplasticity

Neuroplasticity is the brain's power to change itself in positive ways. Think of the brain as being like malleable plastic. If we repeatedly bring change to our normal routines, our brain is forced to remould itself, to activate new patterns of thinking and carve out new neural pathways.

The neuroscience of the brain's left and right hemispheres is complicated, but we do know that stimulating activity across both hemispheres via the brain's communication centre, the **corpus callosum**, stimulates neural connections, particularly when we change the way we perform basic tasks – using our non-preferred hand, for example. Doing the same things the same ways all the time can be extremely beneficial to us, but it can also lead to thinking patterns or habits that do not help us.

Our sleep (or lack thereof) is highly patterned and habitual. We need to change the pattern. How quickly can we do that with some simple, repetitive changes that may occur in our lives?

If we keep stimulating new associations we will continue to improve our brain function, and this applies to trying to get an even better sleep. Doing these sorts of activities means we use more parts of our brain, which may also create opportunities to find solutions to problems that are nagging us and interrupting our sleep.

If we repeatedly bring change to our normal routines, we activate new patterns of thinking.

EXERCISE
Change hands

Colour in the drawing below (or a copy of it) using your *non-writing hand*. This stimulates the neurons in the opposite hemisphere and encourages neuroplasticity.

Time to go through the colouring techniques you've already learned. Put your earphones in, pick a colour you relate to today, and colour in with your non-preferred hand until the alpha sounds stop.

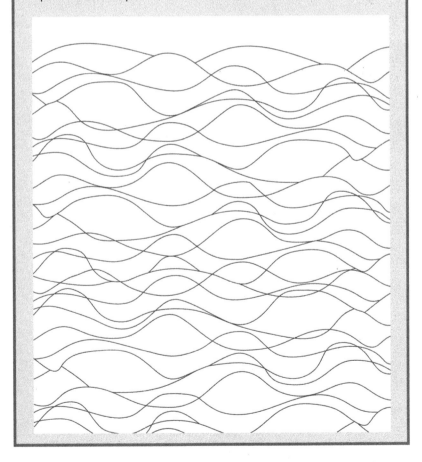

EXERCISE
The infinity symbol

Using your writing hand, trace over the infinity symbol above with a pen or pencil. Practise a few times.

When you feel like you have the knack of it, fill the rest of this page (or a blank piece of paper) with infinity symbols.

Now place the pen or pencil in your other (non-writing) hand. Fill the rest of this page (or a blank piece of paper) with the infinity symbol.

It may be a little awkward to begin with, but persevere and it will get easier.

continued

In this final part of the exercise, put a pen or pencil in *each hand*.

At the same time, side by side, draw *two infinity symbols*. Try to start both symbols at different points, and move both hands in opposite directions.

You are now stimulating both your right and left brain hemispheres, to enable better neuroplasticity.

EXERCISE

Square, circle, triangle

Using your writing hand, trace over the three shapes above with a pen or pencil. Practise a few times.

When you feel like you have the knack of it, fill the rest of this page and the next (or a blank piece of paper) with the three shapes.

continued

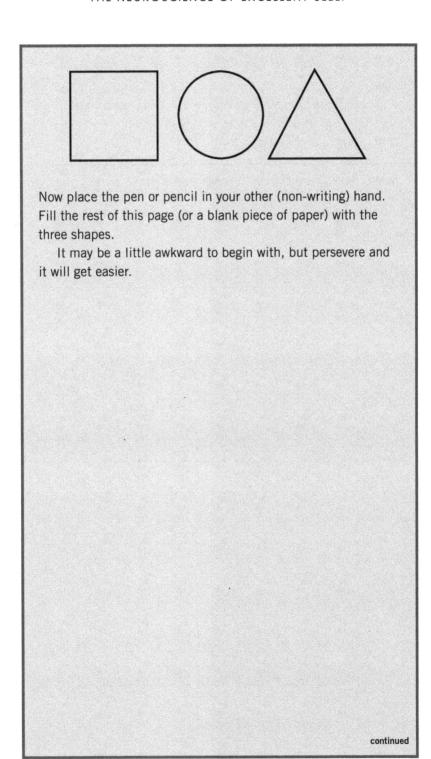

Now place the pen or pencil in your other (non-writing) hand. Fill the rest of this page (or a blank piece of paper) with the three shapes.

It may be a little awkward to begin with, but persevere and it will get easier.

continued

In this final part of the exercise, put a pen or pencil in *each hand*.

At the same time, side by side, draw *two of the three shapes*. Try to start both shapes at different points, and move both hands in opposite directions.

You are now stimulating both your right and left brain hemispheres, to enable better neuroplasticity.

EXERCISE

Change everyday things around

You can change a lot of the everyday things you do in order to help your brain start thinking in different ways. Try doing this in the morning to get your brain fired up for the day – for example, brushing your teeth with your non-dominant hand (including opening the tube and applying the toothpaste). You could substitute any morning activity (as long as it's not potentially dangerous): styling or brushing your hair, applying face cream, eating breakfast. You could also use only one hand to do tasks like buttoning a shirt. When you can, try using just your non-preferred hand.

Another exercise that associates unusual sensory and motor pathways in your cortex with a routine activity is using *your feet* to put your socks and underwear in the laundry basket, or pick out your shoes for the day.

Using the hand you don't normally favour stimulates the neurons in the opposite hemisphere of the brain and encourages neuroplasticity.

BRAIN EXERCISES TO USE BEFORE OR AFTER SLEEP

It's just as important to prepare our brain for sleep as it is to prepare it for each new day. The following exercises build on the brain exercises we've done during the day by relaxing our brain and body at night, and waking them up fully in the morning.

Engaging our senses

As we saw in **A MULTI-SENSORY TECHNIQUE FOR EXCELLENT SLEEP** (pages 73 to 80), using one or more of our five senses is the perfect way to relax our brain. Our senses are the means by which the brain receives all its information. These connections are very strong and the neural pathways created by them are deeply embedded. If we want to change our thinking, we need to utilise these deep connections to help create calming thoughts.

Sight and touch

Most of us understand the power of being **tactile**. That touch, kiss, hug or simple pat on the shoulder registers very quickly with us, particularly with our brain. Our **sight** is also a strong sensory trigger linked to our spatial memory.

Many parts of our brain are suppressed when we rely on our eyes. Think about the things you do before bed that are linked to your sight. If you try to do them with your eyes closed, you will stimulate very rarely used brain circuits, and allow your brain to create new associations with these tasks. If you close your eyes and use only the power of touch, your hands will probably notice different textures on your own body that you're not even aware of when your eyes are open. This will enable you to shake off bad patterns and find new pathways to better, even *excellent*, sleep.

EXERCISE
Close your eyes

Try to do the things you normally do before bed with your eyes closed. Get undressed, rearrange the covers, turn out the lights and perform all your other bedtime rituals – all without sight. Of course, you need to be careful – don't try anything that may be dangerous.

EXERCISE
Close your eyes in the shower

In the shower, locate the taps and adjust the temperature and flow using just your tactile senses. Then wash, shave and so on, all with your eyes shut. Make sure your balance is good and the shower is not too slippery before you try this and, again, be careful: use common sense to avoid burning or injury.

This exercise is quick and easy to do, and very good for free-flow thinking and problem-solving. Have a shower before bed, close your eyes and let your brain come up with ideas or solutions to any problems that are troubling you.

EXERCISE
Get more tactile

When you get dressed in the morning, without looking, choose clothing, shoes and so on that have matching or contrasting textures. Use not only your fingers but also your cheeks, lips and even your feet – they're all packed with sensitive receptors, allowing for fine responses. Try this when you get changed before bed too, and learn to associate the experience with relaxation.

Sound

How many times in the morning do you find yourself only half
awake and half listening? You hear a couple of words and off
you go, completing the sentence before you hear any more.
The brain is really good at tuning in and out like this, but it
means that it remains sluggish and doesn't wake up properly.

Helping our brain to achieve an *excellent sleep* involves
creating **a clearer distinction between being asleep and
being awake**. (This is also the theory behind my **DECAF
NAPPUCCINO** brain-stretching exercises on pages 85 to 105.)

EXERCISE
Waking up the brain

Try wearing earplugs when you join the family for breakfast and
experience the world without sound. This will quickly train your
brain to wake up and be alert. Most importantly, it will help you
learn to distinguish between being asleep and awake, which is
critical to achieving *excellent sleep*.

Smell

The brain's ability to change itself works particularly well with
regard to smell. The brain's olfactory bulb, which interacts
with the hippocampus and the amygdala as required, makes
strong smell-related associations, such as a particular
perfume with a mother or partner, or roast dinner with family.

EXERCISE
Smell something different

To change your usual morning olfactory associations – such as enjoying the smell of freshly brewed coffee – wake up to something different, such as vanilla, citrus or peppermint tea.

For *excellent sleep*, keep an extract of the aroma you associate with relaxation in an airtight container on your bedside table and release the scent into the air before bed. Your brain will soon associate that odour with your need for sleep.

This is a particularly good technique for those who need to sleep in different places. The association of the aroma with the act of sleep rather than with your bedroom can get you sleeping far more quickly and deeply.

Engaging ALL our senses

For many of us, showers are the norm and baths are for our young children, or for when we have the time – which is usually very rarely indeed. From a neuroscience perspective, this is a misjudgment, because a warm bath has tremendous sensory power. Our skin, which is our body's largest organ, is covered in sensory stimulus receptors that immediately relax when we immerse ourselves in hot water.

EXERCISE
Multi-sensory stimulation at bath time

Try to create a multi-sensory bath-time experience by lighting scented candles, adding bath oils to the water, listening to your favourite music, drinking camomile tea or just one small glass of champagne, and using sponges, body scrubs and plush towels. This will create strong associations with relaxation for the brain.

Try extending these associations to your bedroom experience. Keep the light in the bathroom at the same level as it is when you go to sleep in your bedroom, as this will strengthen the new linkages in the brain. Use the same scented candles or music when you go to bed and the brain will automatically create all the associations you experienced while luxuriating in your bath.

Bedtime neuroplasticity

We learned on page 96 that switching our everyday routines around will encourage our brain's neuroplasticity – its ability to change itself by creating new neural pathways. While it's extremely important to have bedtime routines to relax us for sleep, the task of achieving *excellent sleep* may mean we have to disturb our existing routines and create new ones that enable us to perform that much better. Our current practices are locking us into achieving the same results all the time. Time to change the brain pathways that may be holding us back.

EXERCISE
Change things around before sleep

Try changing your routines, just a little, before sleep. Read for a shorter period, and do some relaxation breathing instead – try the 'Micro-break breathing' exercise on page 90. Or put your book away and just listen to relaxing music.

Check in the morning to see how you feel. Go outside and take some deep breaths of fresh air.

Experiment with new activities and adjust your brain patterns to get an even better sleep.

EXERCISE
Sleep on the other side of the bed

Push the boundaries of your habits by learning to sleep *anywhere* – starting with the other side of the bed. This unfamiliar position will activate your hippocampus and cortex to integrate the new feelings you experience by sleeping in a different position. The brain literally creates a new map, allowing you to reach a new destination: *better sleep*.

SELF-HYPNOSIS EXERCISES FOR EXCELLENT SLEEP

We learned in **Part 2** about the serious impact stress can have not just on our sleep, but also on our health in general. When someone is under extreme pressure at home or work, to help their body perform better they can either remove the stress from their life or find ways to cope with it.

Certain life situations are very difficult, such as the chronic illness of oneself or a loved one. Since this situation will remain constant until the person gets well or dies, the only recourse is to learn strategies to lessen the effects of this perpetual stress upon the body. If we find ourselves in such a situation, **self-hypnosis** is a technique we can use to manage our thoughts and emotions.

When the stressful situation is due to work, relationships or other transient factors, the best approach is to change the situation. But while someone *outside* the situation may see this as easy, when we're immersed in it numerous beliefs and emotions can prevent us from seeing the possibilities of change available to us. Self-hypnosis can assist us in these circumstances too, by addressing our limiting beliefs and overcoming the fear that is immobilising us. Once we're out of the stressful situation, our body can marshal its forces to come back into balance, or homeostasis.

Let's look firstly at how we can use self-hypnosis to affect our sleep.

The Excellent Sleep Mindset

All forms of hypnosis are in fact *self*-hypnosis, because none of us can simply be told to do something we don't want to do. The key is getting ourselves into a meditative or trance-like state, a state in which we become highly open to suggestions.

This state is not wakefulness and not sleep, but something in between. In neuroscience terms, it's referred as the **alpha–theta state**, and is very similar to Stage 1 of sleep (page 35). For many of us it lasts just a few minutes, but it can extend to up to half an hour. It is during this period of relaxation that we can access the brain's habitual thought pathways and introduce them to other thoughts, desires and goals – such as better sleep.

To cultivate an Excellent Sleep Mindset, during this suggestive period we need to imagine ourselves feeling comfortable, safe and fast asleep. If we do this often enough, the quantity and quality of our sleep will begin to come into line with our wishes, thanks to the principles of neuroplasticity. Later, we'll apply the same technique to many areas of our life that can affect our sleep, such as our surroundings, health problems, sleep disorders and the anxieties we experience each day.

Neuroscience research shows that self-hypnosis can significantly relax and de-stress the mind and body. Alpha–theta brain activity is increasingly being shown to protect the immune system from the negative effects of stress, and this protection is boosted by *excellent sleep*.

We can practise self-hypnosis techniques daily, or as often as we feel the need. Of course, long-lasting changes to our sleep patterns are best achieved by using a daily routine that involves an Excellent Sleep Mindset.

The following brain routine should start to show results in as little as a few days to a week.

Ensure you are in a calm and relaxed state, in which your goal is *excellent sleep*. As you repeat the words of the Excellent Sleep Mindset each night, your brain will begin to take these ideas on board and treat them as real. In fact, the subconscious brain treats *all* thoughts as real, even if they are not. Soon these thoughts will grow familiar and comfortable. The key is repeated practice.

EXERCISE
The Excellent Sleep Routine

1. Get into bed and get comfortable. Make sure you've got all the basics right for *excellent sleep* (see pages 67 to 72).

2. Read the Excellent Sleep Mindset, either aloud or to yourself:

I will find that each night from now on I will have an EXCELLENT SLEEP. I will sleep soundly and peacefully, for the length of time I need. I can imagine myself in a state of deep relaxation, in which my chest is rhythmically moving up and down. I can picture myself deeply asleep.

I will shortly become drowsy. I will fall asleep as soon as I put this book down and close my eyes. If I wake during the night, I will very quickly slip back into a deep sleep, with

continued

pleasant dreams that will help me sort out my problems. On the rare occasions when I do lie awake and find it difficult to sleep, the time will seem to pass quickly and I will find ways to put this time to good use. When the number of hours available is not sufficient for excellent sleep, *the sleep I do have will be more effective. Every hour will feel like more, and in the morning I will wake up refreshed and alert.*

I will get drowsy and fall asleep as soon as I finish my Excellent Sleep Routine.

3. Find a point to focus on and fix your gaze on it. Take a deep breath in and hold it for a moment, then breathe out slowly, as we practised earlier in the book ('Micro-break breathing', page 90). As you do so, silently repeat to yourself:
'My eyelids are heavy and ready to close, I can relax and let go.' Say this to yourself a few times, then close your eyes and relax.

4. Breathe in and out slowly and count down from five to zero: '5 ... 4 ... 3 ... 2 ... 1 ... 0.' Tell yourself that with every count, you're becoming more relaxed. Focus on your breathing and how relaxed your body is becoming.

5. Stay in this relaxed state for a few minutes. During this time, calmly and confidently state your desire for *excellent sleep,* either in your mind or out loud. Repeat the suggestion a few times and just feel it wash over you. If you want to, you can also visualise yourself in a beautiful, deep sleep.

6. Repeat this each night, remembering to be patient with yourself. Being excellent at anything takes time, and achieving *excellent sleep* is no different.

Note: If you have trouble achieving a state of relaxation then replace steps 4 and 5 with listening to **binaural beats technology** (page 77) for thirty minutes before sleep. This will enable your brain to achieve a pre-sleep alpha state conducive to the Excellent Sleep Mindset.

More self-hypnosis messages for *excellent sleep*

When things are on our mind – consciously or unconsciously – we can find ourselves having difficulty sleeping. Each of the messages below deals with a different problem that may be impeding our sleep.

Sometimes our external environment is preventing us from getting a good night's sleep. Sometimes it is a health issue or sleep disorder. And sometimes the things that are affecting our sleep are going on in our daily lives and we just can't stop thinking about them.

Simply use the exercise on pages 115 to 116 and replace the Excellent Sleep Mindset with the message below that is relevant to you. They can all be used in conjunction with **binaural beats technology**, especially if you find it particularly difficult to focus, or you want to achieve an even deeper state of relaxation.

If *your* particular issue isn't included here, why not write your own version of the Excellent Sleep Mindset?

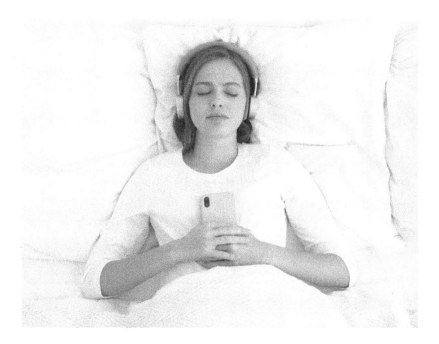

EXERCISE
Difficulties sleeping due to noise sensitivity

From now on, when I am in bed my perception of outside noise will be altered. The sounds I once heard as loud and annoying will become fainter and softer, fading further and further away. From now on, I will be aware of these sounds but they simply won't bother me. They will flow over me, over and away and into the distance. They will be remote and quite unimportant. I will remain calm and detached. Calm and detached. From now on, my unconscious mind will return my sound sensitivity to a level where I will not be bothered by outside noise at all.

EXERCISE
Difficulties with sleeping due to sleepwalking

When I sleep I will rarely find it necessary to get out of bed during the night, unless I am completely awake and aware of what is happening around me. From now on, I will sleep peacefully and soundly when I am in bed, dreaming constructive, pleasant dreams, and it will be difficult to disturb me. If I get out of bed when I am not awake, the moment my feet touch the ground, I will wake up and become aware of what is happening.

EXERCISE
Difficulties sleeping due to light sensitivity

From now on, that part of me that has been paying far too much attention to the amount of light in the room, that part of me that has been irritated and upset by the room's light, is going to pay less and less attention to that light. I will still be aware that the lighting is there, and that sometimes the lights appear to flicker a little or are too bright. But I will cease to pay very much attention to this light, just as if that part of me was extremely alert before but has now become dulled, unable to devote much attention to any light in the room. I will be able to settle and prepare to sleep without noticing the light very much, as if it has become further away. This light simply won't bother me any more.

EXERCISE
Difficulties with sleeping due to tinnitus

From now on, I will pay less and less attention to the noises in my ears. They will recede into the distance, becoming fainter and fainter. Further and further away. They will flow over and away from me. I will be less and less sensitive to these noises. Soon they will bother me very, very little. Instead, when I settle down to sleep at night, my unconscious mind will fill my brain with my favourite sounds. It will seem as if I can actually hear my favourite sounds being played in my head as I drift off to sleep.

EXERCISE

Difficulties with socialising and communicating

From now on, I will find it easier to appear confident. I will work at presenting myself as self-assured. Gradually I will actually become the way I want to appear. In social situations I will be much less self-conscious, less preoccupied with myself, much less concerned about other people's opinions of me.

From now on, I will be more outgoing and friendly with people. I will choose my words more and more skilfully. I will be able to talk quite confidently with strangers at a party. I will concentrate on other people and show genuine interest in them – what they are doing and how they are feeling. I will ask them questions and really listen to the answers. I will accept compliments gracefully and pay other people compliments in return. I will look them in the eye when I talk to them, smile readily, look approachable. I will be prepared to go more than halfway when making friendly overtures to other people, and be prepared for rejection. It will hurt less and less as time goes by. Teasing remarks will have less and less effect on me. I will realise they are being said more in fun than with the intention of upsetting or hurting me.

From now on, I will read as widely as possible, and expand my activities and my circle of acquaintances. I will make a mental note of interesting things I have read or done, short funny jokes, and anything else I could use as a conversation item. But I will also be prepared to be silent. I don't have to try to fill gaps in conversation all the time.

I will be more adventurous where making friends is concerned and much more outgoing. My confidence will increase steadily, day by day. My mind will be clearer and I will be able to speak up and express my opinions easily.

EXERCISE

Difficulties with assertiveness

From now on, I will become more and more assertive, more able to stand up for myself without undue anxiety, to express my honest feelings comfortably and to obtain my rights without interfering with the rights of others. I will act firmly by speaking up if someone is served out of turn in front of me in a shop or if the food is unsatisfactory in a restaurant. If someone asks me a favour I do not wish to grant, I will simply say, 'I'm sorry, but no.' I will be able to assert myself more and more in situations I would once have found difficult to handle. In being assertive, I will also become sensitive to the feelings of others, so that my relationships will be mutually satisfying. The more assertive and spontaneous I become, the more confident I will feel, the better I will feel about myself and the more other people will respect and admire me.

Neuroscience research shows that self-hypnosis can significantly relax and de-stress the mind and body.

EXERCISE
Difficulty with anger

From now on, I will be able to get in touch with my pent-up emotions and deal with them in a constructive manner. Whenever similar feelings are directed against me, I will find acceptable ways to redirect them. Perhaps I will imagine myself beating a pillow with my fists until all those angry feelings inside me have evaporated, beating it harder and harder until I am completely exhausted, yelling and screaming in my mind until I am too worn out and tired to go on.

Maybe I will redirect it towards some positive, constructive purpose. Or I will climb up into a dusty old attic in my mind where all the outdated things are kept, all the things that no longer have a useful purpose to serve. I will take off my past hurts, anger and bitterness like an old, worn-out coat, and leave them behind in the attic, locking the door as I leave.

All the hidden personal reasons for my angry, hostile feelings may or may not be communicated to my conscious mind. The awareness that IS communicated to my conscious mind will be dealt with in a constructive, practical and sensible way. Whatever still remains of these feelings that is no longer serving any useful purpose will be dumped by my unconscious mind down an imaginary laundry chute, leaving me quite free to get on with my life.

EXERCISE
Difficulty with guilt

From now on, my mind will start to process my guilty feelings at all levels. It will gradually accept that because I am only human, I have human failings. That I have made mistakes and done things I should not have done, and not done things I should have done. At times I have been careless or irresponsible, and at times I have hurt others and myself.

My unconscious mind will especially dwell on ways of safely dealing with the guilt that I have repressed from an early age, concerning jealousy of and anger at other people. My unconscious mind will find ways of accepting and assimilating these things and seeing that they are of no importance. At all levels, my mind will begin to come to terms with and discard those guilty feelings I have no control over – guilts from the past that I can no longer do anything about. I will shake them off completely, at all levels. My mind will also work on ways to get rid of more recent guilty feelings, by taking action to change what can be changed and to make up somehow for what I have done or left undone in the present or the recent past.

EXERCISE
Difficulty with feeling low and flat

From now on, when I start to feel flat or low, I will immediately distract myself with plans, ideas or activities. I will quickly recover my sense of humour and my sense of proportion. I will feel better and more optimistic, and have renewed energy. I will dwell on the things I am grateful for, on happy memories and on the things I have to look forward to.

I won't get nearly so upset about teasing remarks or hurtful incidents. These will have less and less effect on me. I will realise that they can't really upset or hurt me. They just won't bother me any more. From now on, when I am slighted or rejected I won't be nearly as hurt. Things just won't be able to get under my skin as much. I may get a little sad, but I won't be devastated. Inwardly I will be much stronger, much better able to withstand hurts and disappointments. I will be far less vulnerable than before.

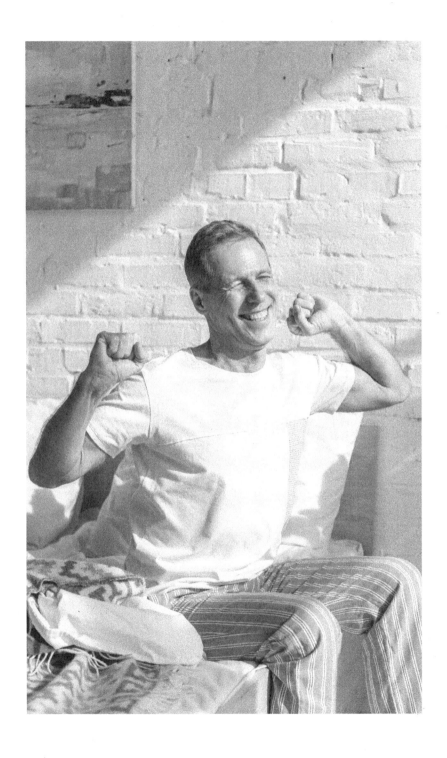

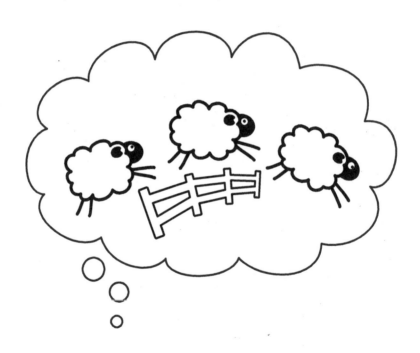

PART 4

CHILDREN AND EXCELLENT SLEEP

'Small children disturb your sleep,
big children your life.'

—Yiddish proverb

MY CHILD HAS A SLEEP PROBLEM – WHAT CAN I DO?

Becoming an *excellent sleeper* ideally begins when we're first brought home from the delivery ward. In this part of the book, I'm going to devote some time to exploring how we can give our babies, children and adolescents the best possible start on the road to a lifetime of *excellent sleep*.

Often our children suffer from sleep disturbances. They just don't seem able to settle themselves at night. They need our help with rocking, holding or talking until they fall asleep.

If only the problems stopped there. During the night they wake several times, crying or calling out, and each time you go in and help them get back to sleep. You're tired and frustrated, and even starting to get angry with them, because *your* sleep has been disturbed too. At the same time you're feeling guilty, because you know they're not waking on purpose, and if they need you, you have to be there.

These problems are extremely common, but can be very frustrating for parents and carers to deal with. Many of us have been told that these difficulties settling and night wakings are normal, and there's nothing to do but wait until they grow out of it. But **this behaviour is not normal**, and **you do not have to wait for things to change**. When a child can't seem to settle down at night, or is generally restless in bed, you should never just assume that they are naturally a poor sleeper, or don't need as much sleep as other children. While sleeping problems are very common, they are usually not inherent.

Your own expectations can have a very profound influence on how your child's sleep patterns develop from the very first day you bring them home from the hospital. If you are led very early to believe that your baby is just a poor sleeper, and there is nothing you can do about it, this allows them to develop bad habits that leave the whole family suffering.

Most of the time, parents and carers can identify the causes of sleep disturbance and successfully bring about the necessary changes. Even when your child is as young as five or six months old, you can begin to solve their sleep problems. If you wait and do nothing, their sleep will eventually improve by itself, but it could take many months or even longer. If you can find out why your child is not sleeping well and take steps to correct the problem, their sleep will usually improve in **less than two weeks**.

It's true that children differ in their ability to sleep. Some are *excellent sleepers* from birth, and may even have to be woken up for their feeds in the early weeks. As they grow older, not only do they continue to sleep well, but it is also difficult to wake them up even if you want to. They sleep soundly at night in a variety of situations – light or dark, quiet or noisy, calm or chaotic. They tolerate occasional disruption of their sleep schedules, and even sleep well during emotionally upsetting situations.

Other children seem inherently more susceptible to having their sleep patterns disrupted. Any change in bedtime routines, any illness, hospital visit or house guest may cause their sleep patterns to become worse. But, just as with us adults, these children will be able to sleep quite satisfactorily once appropriate changes are made to their routines, schedules, surroundings and interactions with family. They may still have occasional nights of poor sleep, but if the new routines continue to be followed consistently, normal patterns of sleep will follow.

There are a very, very few children who will continue to sleep poorly for unknown reasons, or reasons that haven't yet been identified. But the great news is that nearly all children without a major medical or neurological disorder are capable of achieving *excellent sleep*. They will be able to go to bed at an appropriate time, fall asleep within minutes, and stay asleep until a reasonable hour in the morning.

When should I worry?

The answer is **when their sleeping patterns cause a problem for you or them**.

Some sleep problems – such as sleep terrors or sleepwalking – are **quite easy to identify**. Others, however, are **less obvious** and you may not even recognise your child even has a problem, or that the problem they have should be treated. Other indicators of possible sleep problems are trouble at bedtime, waking during the night and not going straight back to sleep, falling asleep too early or too late, waking too early or too late in the morning, or being irritable or sleepy during the day.

Let's start by looking at **what happens when children sleep**, just as we did for adult sleep. This will give you a good idea of what *should* be happening, so you can start to identify any potential problems with your own child's sleep habits. The next priority is to **find the best daily schedule** for your child. As we'll discover, discrepancies in this area can lead to problems in so many others. Then we'll deal one by one with the major things that could be going wrong with your child's sleep:

1. Problems with **getting to sleep**

2. Problems with **waking during the night**

3. Problems with **their biological clock**

4. Problems involving **lost sleep**.

So read on to find out how, in a relatively short space of time, you and your child can go from bedroom woes and worries to *excellent sleep* …

Nearly all children without a major medical or neurological disorder are capable of achieving excellent sleep.

WHAT HAPPENS WHEN CHILDREN SLEEP

We've already looked in some detail at the brain's behaviour during sleep in **Part 2**, but what I'd like to do now is look more specifically at the child's brain. We can see how the brain develops, particularly over the first six months of life, by looking at the **changing stages and patterns of children's sleep**.

Unborn babies

There is significant evidence to show that sleep patterns begin to develop in babies even before birth.

The earliest stage to form is **REM sleep**. It appears in the foetus at about **six or seven months' gestation**, and **non-REM sleep** between **seven and eight months**. By the end of the eighth month of gestation, both states are well established, but the unborn infant's non-REM sleep **has not yet divided into four stages**.

In the foetus and infant (up to three months), REM sleep is referred to as **Active Sleep** and non-REM as **Quiet Sleep**. Active Sleep is most important in the early months as the foetus develops. This preponderance of Active Sleep in the early stages of development is not fully understood, but we do know that Quiet Sleep requires a certain degree of brain maturation, which we wouldn't expect to see in the foetus or newborn. We of course know nothing of foetus or infant 'dreams'; Active Sleep may allow the baby's developing brain to receive sensory input even before birth. This input may be important to the development of the higher, most sophisticated brain centres that are involved in thought, such as the frontal cortex.

The baby in the uterus makes no breathing motions in Quiet Sleep, but does make them in Active Sleep. If respiratory movements were never practised, the child would be born with no experience at all in using these muscles that are so vital to survival. It is conceivable that the unborn baby is also practising sending out signals that control other motor activity. We learned earlier (pages 12 and 40) that the motor cortex, which controls the body's movement, is switched off in adults during REM sleep; the same applies to children. In the foetus this area is not so completely blocked, so there is some actual ability to practise body movements during Active (REM) Sleep.

Newborn babies

While **sixteen or seventeen hours' sleep per day** is the norm for newborn babies, they are unable to sleep for more than a few hours at a time. As a result, they will have about **seven sleeping and waking periods**, evenly distributed throughout the day and night. The sleep periods will vary from twenty minutes to six hours. Even when the baby sleeps well for a few hours, you can easily observe brief arousals.

Unlike children and adults, the newborn enters **Active Sleep** immediately after falling asleep. This sleep stage is easy to identify because the baby twitches and breathes irregularly, and you can see their eyes dart about under their thin eyelids.

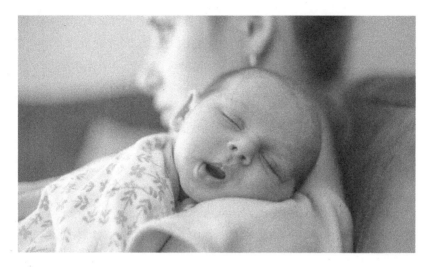

Sometimes you may also see a brief smile. Premature babies spend **80 per cent** of their sleep time in this state and full-term infants **50 per cent**.

In **Quiet Sleep**, the baby breathes deeply and lies very still. Occasionally you may see fast sucking motions, and now and then a sudden body jerk. While the Quiet Sleep stage is well formed in newborn infants, it is still somewhat different from the non-REM sleep of older children and us adults (pages 37 and 40). The brain waves during this stage show large, slow waves, occurring in bursts rather than in a continuous flow.

During the first month, the non-REM brain waves become continuous and the jerks and starts disappear. By one month of age, **sleep spindles** (page 36) begin to appear, and over the next month **a sequence of non-REM sleep stages** becomes identifiable. We do not see the **K-complex** waves (page 36) until about six months of age.

Three-month-old babies

Over the first three months, most infants begin to adjust on their own to the external cues of light, noise and activity during the day, and darkness, quiet and lack of activity at night, by developing **a well-formed rhythm of approximately**

twenty-four hours. By three months old – four at the latest – they are sleeping about **fifteen hours a day**. By this age some children have also **settled** – that is, they are getting most of their sleep at night, usually in a continuous episode of **five to nine hours**. They continue to nap at **three or four** fairly predictable times of the day and have one or more periods of prolonged waking.

By this time, **non-REM sleep** has developed all four distinct stages. The sleep pattern will have consolidated into about **four or five** sleep periods, with roughly **60 per cent** of the sleep occurring at night.

Instead of going straight into **REM sleep**, by about three months of age infants will enter non-REM first, something that will continue for the rest of their life. A young child will plunge rapidly through drowsiness and the lighter stages of non-REM sleep into Stage 4, usually within ten minutes.

This pattern will remain fairly constant throughout their life – **hence the need to get these things right early**.

Children six months old and up

By around **six months** of age, nearly all infants will have settled, and continuous night-time sleep will have increased. Typically, a baby of this age will sleep about **twelve hours** at night, with only occasional brief wakings. As you would expect, the pattern of settling varies with each child; some settle in a very erratic fashion, but at some point between three and six months old they should be sleeping well at night. They will commonly also take **two one- to two-hour naps** each day, one mid-morning and a second in the afternoon.

At **one year** of age, most children will sleep **fourteen hours** altogether. If they still have a morning nap, they will almost certainly give it up at some point during the second year.

By **age two**, they should sleep about **eleven to twelve hours** at night, with **a one- to two-hour nap** after lunch. They will continue their nap until at least age three and even up to age five.

From **age three to adolescence**, children need gradually less sleep. After age three, napping is rare. Night-time sleep slowly decreases from around **twelve hours** between **ages three and five** to about **ten hours** between ages **nine and twelve**.

During the years of **puberty** – beginning anywhere from age eight to thirteen in girls and nine to fifteen in boys – rapid changes occur, both physical and psychological. Children aged **fourteen to seventeen** sleep only about seven to eight hours, although, as we will see, the science suggests this is more culturally imposed. As shown in the table of recommended sleep hours on page 15, this group should *actually* be getting **eight to nine hours' sleep** a night.

The following chart sets out the average sleep hours at different times of the day for each age group from newborns to late adolescents.

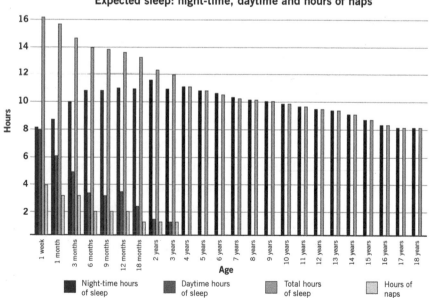

Expected sleep: night-time, daytime and hours of naps

The total amount of **REM sleep** decreases throughout childhood and levels out in adolescence. Although at birth a full-term baby will have **50 per cent** of its sleep in the REM state, only **33 per cent** of sleep will be in REM by age three, and the typical adult level of **20 per cent** will be reached by later childhood or adolescence.

The total amount of **Stage 4 non-REM sleep** also decreases throughout childhood and adolescence as total sleep decreases, but it continues to account for **20 to 25 per cent** of the child's total sleep. In children, Stages 3 and 4 are less distinct than in adults.

The following chart shows the typical sleep pattern of children from three years old to adolescence.

Typical sleep pattern for children

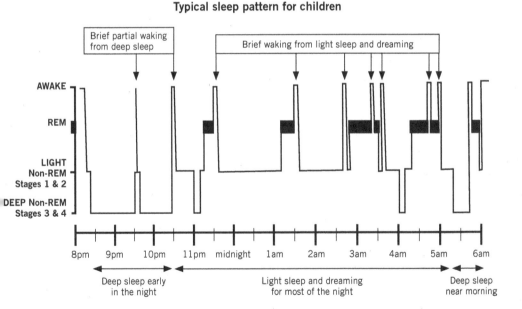

FINDING THE BEST DAILY SCHEDULE

Most infants will develop a good twenty-four-hour sleep schedule in spite of us, but we can help them develop these patterns. To do so we need to take into account the child's habits, learned associations and nutritional and emotional needs, while avoiding approaches that could interfere with the development of their normal rhythms. Try to establish a reasonable daytime schedule for your baby in their first three months and maintain it throughout their childhood. (As we'll see on pages 190 to 203, this is particularly important when it comes to sorting out problems with **children's biological clocks**.)

The first three months

Newborns do not have good patterns of sleep. A baby's sleep pattern during the first few days after birth should not be considered a predictor of things to come. Regardless of whether they sleep well or fitfully in hospital, and of the advice you're given by nurses about their sleep performance, things will inevitably change once they arrive home. If issues do develop, the likely culprit will be the parents' inexperience.

While these issues are frustrating, with time your child will settle into a reasonable schedule.

Mostly they will start to develop a sleep pattern over the **first two weeks**, with many naps – some brief, some longer – distributed across the day and night. As mentioned earlier, some babies seem to sleep unusually well from the start, but this is the exception rather than the rule.

Occasionally they will have their longest sleep period during the day and their longest period of being awake at night. Things seem to be the wrong way around, but this will change. At this age it's impressive that they can display *any* consistent pattern, since they've had little opportunity to form regular daily rhythms, and little or no opportunity to distinguish between day and night. It should be easy to readjust this schedule if they don't do so on their own.

If a pattern develops whereby they are awake much of the night and sleeping as much as six hours at a time during the day, then begin waking them earlier and earlier from the long sleep period, so that you start to treat it as a nap, and move into longer segments during the night. Although you are following their cues to a point, you can still help structure their sleep–wake cycle.

Keep an eye on their periods of activity, feeding, waking and sleep, so that you can anticipate their needs and know when to play with them, feed them or put them down to sleep. While you can't tie their feeds, play and sleep precisely to the clock, if you are aware of their emerging schedule you can encourage them to sleep and eat at reasonable and consistent times during the day. This will further help to stabilise their developing twenty-four-hour cycles.

It usually takes **six to ten weeks** for them to develop a good twenty-four-hour schedule, with the longest period of sleep occurring at night.

Feeding patterns

Feeding patterns are an important part of the infant's daily schedule. It is no longer standard practice to urge parents to put their babies on a precise four-hourly feeding regime from the beginning. Only if they are premature, or have medical problems or feeding difficulties, will you need to follow a rigid feeding schedule.

If your baby has none of these issues, you should **follow their own cues**. But there are problems to watch for in a feeding-on-demand schedule. Firstly, not all cries are hunger cries, and it will take you a little time to discern which sounds mean what.

Secondly, you should only follow your baby's cues *within limits*. A newborn usually needs to be fed **every two to six hours**. Naturally, if they only cry for feeds every twelve hours, something is wrong. They simply have to be fed more often. Even if they are not crying for a feed, they may be ready to feed at the expected time and you'll probably be able to nurse them quite easily.

What may be less readily apparent is that a full-term healthy infant does not need **hourly feeds**, even if they seem hungry this often. Hourly feeding is exhausting for everyone and greatly interferes with their development of healthy sleeping, waking and feeding patterns. If you have been feeding them every hour, begin to increase the time between feeds by an amount you are comfortable with. Try **fifteen or even thirty minutes each day** until you are feeding your child every two, three or even five hours as desired. To do this you may have to tolerate some crying, and find ways to calm them other than food.

This table shows how you might gradually reduce the size of feeds while increasing the time between them.

DAY	Minutes of breast- or bottle-feeding	Hours (minimum) between feeds
1	7	2
2	6	2.5
3	5	3
4	4	3.5
5	3	4
6	2	4.5
7	1	5
8	0	0

Your baby has been born into a good and caring world, and it's only natural that you would want to show them this by responding to their cries for food and trying to do whatever is necessary to calm them. But helping them develop good schedules is an *equally* important part of caring for them. They will stop crying if they are walked, rocked or stroked for a while, and sometimes will even go off to sleep without a feed. After a short time they will adapt to the new schedule and the hourly crying will cease.

Beyond three months

As we've seen, most infants should have settled fully by around three months of age (six months at the latest). This is good for you too, because you will have more time to spend with them during the day. Still, you should keep working with them to further stabilise their schedule.

For the most part, in the early weeks you are following the child's cues, but by three months it becomes very important for you to provide increasingly consistent structure. When you have established a fairly predictable twenty-four-hour pattern, you will need to provide **a consistent routine** from day to day so that those rhythms are maintained. If the times of feeds, play, bath and anything else you do with them are constantly changing, the chances of achieving regular rhythms will be low.

To help them sleep better, it's critical to continue the new schedule rigorously for **several weeks** after they have begun sleeping well. At this point you can start to alter the daytime routine a little. You can eliminate naps occasionally for a special reason, or take them out in the afternoon even though they may fall asleep in the pram, stroller or car.

Keeping to reasonable schedules as much as possible will enable them to develop and maintain good rhythms of sleeping and waking, activity and rest, and hunger and eating. The more regular *their* schedule is, the more *you* will be able to stay on top of the demands of *your* life – of which there are no doubt many.

Infants cannot be expected to maintain a schedule on their own. You will have to set a reasonable one for them and be willing to enforce it. A degree of flexibility will always be required. Some children need more sleep than others, and some are better able to tolerate fluctuations in their day-to-day routines. It is up to you to learn from experience what schedule is best for your child and how hard you need to work to keep to it.

Even after they've settled into a good sleep–wake pattern, it will always be open to **disruption**. There are just so many things that can do this. Teething, illness, travel and an upset in the family can all affect sleep patterns. The key is that you need to intervene if the disruption goes on too long. Restabilise the schedule, help them get rid of any new bad habits and deal with any anxiety if you can.

Consistency around schedules is so important in dealing with sleep problems and achieving *excellent sleep*. If your child is having sleep problems, regardless of age or cause, a schedule will help immensely.

We're now going to look one by one at the major things that can go wrong with your child's sleep, and what you can do about each of them.

Keeping to reasonable schedules
as much as possible will enable children
to develop and maintain good rhythms
of sleeping and waking.

PROBLEM 1:
GETTING TO SLEEP

Nearly all families experience bedtime struggles at one time or another. Children will stall with requests for water, stories, television, time on digital devices, lights on, room checked for monsters, or even 'Can I sleep in your bed?' They will often choose bedtime to initiate fights with siblings.

Once in bed they may appear restless, rolling all over the bed or getting out of bed as they attempt to avoid their worrying thoughts through physical activities.

The period of transition from evening activity to bedtime is very difficult for many children, so it's not surprising that they can be reluctant to go to sleep. As we're about to see, bedtime is all about **separation** and **loss of control**.

Bedtime fears

All of us at some time have felt frightened as we go to sleep at night. For many children this is certainly the case occasionally, and for a few frequently. These fears are very much dependent on their age and stage of emotional and physical development.

Younger children

As they grow, younger children will face many challenges. They must learn to deal with **separation** when you leave them with other people or at daycare or kindy, or even just when you leave the room. And of course, they need to learn to accept the separation from you each night when they fall asleep.

They also need to learn to **control** their behaviour. Curbing feelings of anger, jealousy and aggression, while learning to give and take when interacting with family and friends, is a vital aspect of growing up.

Specific events may intensify anxieties at any time in a child's development. During **toilet training** there are many worries. The child may be resistant to being trained and tempted to soil themselves. However, at the same time they want to please you and may fear your response. Many toddlers find these worries are heightened at night. Going to sleep means relaxing control, so how can they avoid wetting or soiling themselves when they go to sleep?

When children first **start school**, their concerns about separation may increase for a while. They may be reluctant to leave your side and not let you part from them at bedtime.

For a slightly older child, a **scary movie** can be particularly frightening. Your five- or six-year-old can be upset by scenes of aggression, particularly when they relate to them personally, such as anger towards a parent, or scenes involving abandonment, for instance kidnapping. The events in these movies can seem very real to them. All children have aggressive fantasies, and most feel guilty about them, but seeing their thoughts acted out on the screen can become a source of great anxiety.

Significant **social stresses** of any kind over which they have little control, like parents fighting, illness, separation,

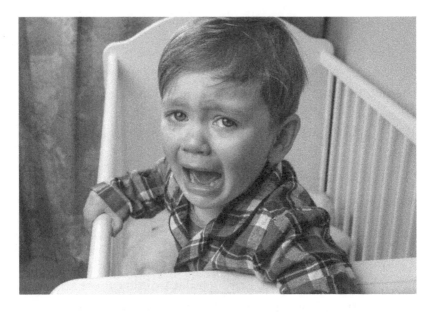

divorce or death, may lead to a great deal of worry, guilt and anxiety at any age. If you were to become ill, for example, they might feel as if their angry thoughts and words have caused your illness.

During the day it's much easier to keep our worries under control. Children keep busy and generally don't have time to brood over their problems. But at night, when they must give up the little control they have over their world, and are unable to continually check their environment, the worrying can begin in earnest. As they get into bed, turn out the lights and lie quietly preparing for sleep, there is little to do but think, and let the fantasies stimulated by their strong feelings run amok.

No wonder bedtime fears and difficulties occur.

Some of the anxieties our children present us with are not realistic. The thought may be that there is a monster in the wardrobe, a goblin under the bed or an intruder outside the window. Although they will be genuinely frightened at these times, they will usually not show overwhelming panic.

As they get sleepy, the ability to avoid certain thoughts decreases. There is less control over feelings, urges and fears.

In this state they begin to feel more childish, and may even act that way. At night, a four- or five-year-old in this state will need the same degree of reassurance as a two- or three-year-old needs during the day. A five-year-old who has no difficulty leaving you for school in the daytime may have much more trouble leaving you to go to sleep at night.

Older children

As children grow towards **adolescence**, they continue to learn, wonder and worry. Their anxieties increase as they mature from children to adults and undergo the rapid physical and emotional changes of **puberty**. Death, God, heaven and hell come into their world and **moral issues** become more relevant. They face constant dilemmas as they try to make many new and important decisions. Like adults, they start to worry about aspects of **their future**, such as leaving school, career and money. While this is going on, they will be experiencing intense **sexual feelings**. They will find pleasure in, but also worry about, genital stimulation.

During all this, they must weigh up peer pressures, personal desires and family standards against issues such as school performance and drug and alcohol use. They must experiment with their new value system while abandoning their existing one. As a parent or carer, you will be continually monitoring your teen against your own expectations while they question their ability to perform against their peers. They may believe you no longer trust or support them, and they may even reject your help completely.

Calming their fears

Whatever your child's age, even if they feel fairly confident that they can take care of themselves in the daytime, at nighttime, when they're less sure of themselves, they will need you to be more involved with them.

Start by laying good foundations for *excellent sleep*. Develop a **bedroom ritual** that includes a special time together each night, to help them get to sleep and stay asleep. Give them a **special object for sleep** that will ease the separation from you at night. Sort out **whose bed** they will sleep in; it will make more difference than you realise. And help them defeat the **monsters in the bedroom** – whether those monsters are literal, or metaphorical. (There are a few other bedtime problems that are specifically to do with **children's biological clocks**; you can read about them later, on pages 190 to 202.)

Bedtime rituals

Bedtime rituals or routines are the activities that take place as you prepare your child for bed and while they fall asleep.

There are many different ways for us to interact with our children at sleep times, and most importantly shape their habits towards *excellent sleep*. These interactions are influenced by **differences within families, ethnic groups and cultures**.

The sleeping child may be tightly bound or swaddled, lightly clothed or even have no clothing on at all. They may sleep in their own room, share a room with one or many, or the entire family may sleep in the same room or even the same bed. The child may go to sleep on their stomach, side or back, in a room that is dark, dimly lit or quite bright. It may be quiet, or there may be occasional noises from aircraft, sirens or other children, or constant sounds such as air conditioners. They may fall asleep while you are nursing them or rocking them in a chair, or alone, perhaps sucking on a pacifier. They may go to sleep only after hearing a bedtime story, praying, playing a quiet game or discussing the day's events. They may go to bed at different times every night, or they may follow exactly the same routine each and every night.

While some bedtime rituals are better than others, there are few **absolute rules** regarding sleep behaviour:

🍂 Your routine must be **working**.

🍂 You and your child must be **happy** with it.

🍂 They must **fall asleep** easily.

🍂 **Night waking** must be infrequent.

🍂 They must be **getting enough sleep**.

🍂 Their **daytime behaviour** must be appropriate.

If all that is the case, then it's likely that whatever you're doing is fine. However, it's important to keep in mind that some routines and approaches are more likely to help develop *excellent sleep* now and avoid problems later in life.

Babies and younger children

When your child is an infant, you probably change their nappy and then hold them until they fall asleep. You then move them to their crib or bed. Or the infant may still be awake when you put them down, so that they fall asleep on their own.

Either of these patterns is fine for the first few months, when you don't expect your baby to sleep through the night anyway. But, as we've just learned, after three months most full-term healthy infants are, or could be, sleeping through the majority of the night. If your baby hasn't **settled by five or six months**, then it's time to take a closer look at their bedtime routine.

If your child is always nursed or rocked to sleep, or if you lie in bed with them till they fall asleep, they may have difficulty going back to sleep alone after normal night-time arousals. Try **putting them to bed awake** so that they can learn to settle themselves and fall asleep alone both at bedtime and after night-time wakings. (Read **Building good associations for *excellent sleep*** [pages 160 to 171] for more detail on this.)

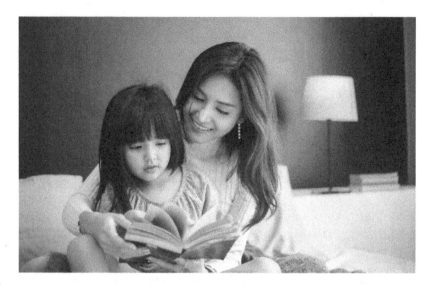

As we've just learned, with children it's important to **follow routines as consistently as you can** – and bedtime is no exception. You should know when they need to change into their pyjamas, brush their teeth and go to bed.

You should choose a routine that suits your family, but always make sure you allow enough time to spend with your child each night before bed. We've just seen that separating from you at night is difficult for children, especially if they're very young. Simply sending a toddler or young child off to bed alone is unfair, even scary. It also means you miss out on what could be one of the best times of the day with them.

Set aside **up to thirty minutes** to do something special with your child before bed. As you would before *your own* bedtime, avoid teasing, scary stories or anything that will excite them. Leave the wrestling for other times of the day. Quiet story-reading and play encourage the brain to enter pre-sleep mode, where brain-wave activity is low.

Children will learn **the rules surrounding this special time** only if you enforce them. They should know what bedtime activities are planned or how many stories will be read, and how much time they will take. Make sure they understand that your time together will not extend beyond the window previously agreed.

It is not a good idea to say when the time is almost up, or when you have only a few pages of the book to go. Don't give in to their pleas for just one more story. If you *both* know what is going to happen, there won't be any of the arguments and tension that arise when there is uncertainty.

Older children

As your child grows older, routines at bedtime continue to be very important. If bedtime is a pleasant time, they will look forward to this part of the day, instead of becoming fussy when it's time for sleep.

They need **close, warm and personal time**. Just watching television together does not achieve this. Even if the show you watch is not exciting or scary, the lack of direct personal interaction makes this bedtime routine a poor choice. Instead, use your special time together to discuss school, plans for the weekend, sport, music lessons and so on. It would also be very helpful during this time to talk over any worries they may have, so they are less likely to brood over them in bed.

As they get older the bedtime ritual **does not have to be the same each night**. A twelve-year-old will want privacy as they get ready for bed, but do stop in to say goodnight and chat for a while. A final routine before bed will still be important, although they can now handle preparing for bed themselves. They might want to listen to music, read or complete some quiet activity before turning out the light.

Special things for sleep

For a young child, falling asleep with a **transitional object** such as a doll, stuffed animal or special blanket far outweighs the benefits of having you lie in bed with them until they fall asleep. These objects will help them accept the night-time

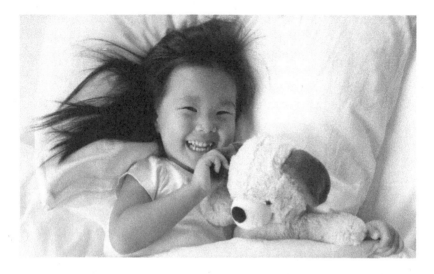

separation from you, and can be a source of reassurance and comfort when they are alone. A special object will give them a feeling of having some control over their world, because they have this object with them whenever they need it, which is something they cannot expect from you. The object will not get up and leave after they fall asleep, and it will be there whenever they wake up.

Children often choose these objects early in their toddler years and may continue to use them up to **age eight**. If your child does not have such a special object, it is reasonable to offer them one that you think may be suitable. However, *they* will always make the final choice, and you cannot *make* them become attached to something. And if you always allow *yourself* to be used in the manner of such an object – to lie with them in bed, to nurse or rock them, to be held, cuddled or even caressed by them, or let them twirl your hair whenever they try to fall asleep – they will never take on a transitional object, because they won't need to.

When they favour a particular object, include it in their bedtime ritual. Have it tucked in next to them, and let it listen to the story or take part in whatever the ritual involves.

Whose bed?

To avoid arguments at bedtime and decrease night-time hassles, many parents give in to their child's desire to share their bed. Some parents feel this is in their child's best interests. Others simply *prefer* to have their child in bed with them.

Although taking a child into bed with you for a night or two may be reasonable if they are ill or very upset about something, for the most part it is **not a good idea**.

We know that **people sleep better alone**. Many studies, including neurological ones, have shown that the movements and arousals of one person during the night stimulate others in the same bed to have more frequent wakings and sleep-state changes, so that they do not sleep as well.

There are even better reasons for *your child* to sleep in their own bed. Sleeping alone is an important part of **learning to separate from you without anxiety and seeing themselves as independent**. This process is important to their psychological and neurological development.

In addition, sleeping in your bed can make them feel confused and anxious rather than relaxed and reassured. Even a young toddler may find this repeated experience over-stimulating. If you allow them to crawl in between you and your partner, in a sense separating the two of you, they may feel too powerful, and become worried. They want **the reassurance of knowing that you are in control**, and that you will do what is best for them regardless of their demands. If the two of you suggest you cannot do this – by letting your child sleep between you – they may become frightened.

If **only one parent is in the bed** then these feelings may in fact be heightened. If you and your partner take the easy way out and allow them into your bed while one of you moves into theirs, they will certainly not be reassured. Now they are *literally* replacing one of you as the other's partner. They may begin to worry that they will cause the two of you to separate, and if this *did* occur they might well feel responsible. Often children of separated or divorced parents feel that *they* caused the family upheaval; they will feel even more confused and unhappy if they have been sleeping in their parent's bed. If as a single parent you begin a new relationship, they will certainly resent being displaced in your bed by this other person.

Nearly all children do not have any serious ongoing problems with sleeping alone. If they are **'too afraid' to do so**, and you deal with this fear by letting them into your bed, you are not really solving the problem. There must be a reason why they are fearful. You will help your child most if you work with them to find and solve the underlying cause of the fear rather than simply letting them sleep with you to ensure a quiet night. This will require patience, understanding and firmness on your part. (See **'Monsters' in the bedroom** [pages 155 to 158] for more detail.)

If **you prefer to have your child in your bed**, you should look at your own feelings very carefully. Some parents

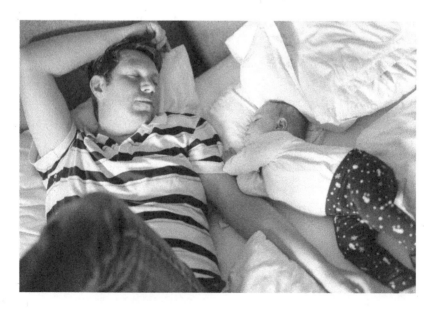

who would otherwise be alone at night find they enjoy the company, feel less lonely, and possibly are less afraid if their child is with them. If there is tension between parents, then taking a child into bed may help avoid confrontation and sexual intimacy. If this is true, then instead of *helping* your child you are *using* them to avoid facing and resolving your own problems. A pattern is formed in which your child and family will suffer. You need to understand and deal with *your own* needs and feelings and resolve the tension between you and your partner.

In the end, if your child always sleeps with you, you may have **great difficulty leaving them**, even with a babysitter. Your social life may be affected, and you may find that you begin to feel resentful of them for this infringement on your life. As they get to the age where you feel they should be sleeping alone, you may find you have **problems moving them into their own bed**.

There are situations in which **they have to sleep with you** for an extended period of time, when living conditions do not permit any other option. You may have only a limited number of bedrooms. Grandparents may be living with you and need a room for themselves. You may be living in someone else's home and only have a single room. Or you may **choose to have your child in your room** for cultural or other reasons.

If they share your bedroom, then make sure they have **their own place to sleep**, such as a cot or a mattress on the floor. Make the corner of the room theirs. Try to have space for some of their things and even a place on the wall for decorations. As soon as you can, move them into a new room, either alone or with sisters and brothers.

'Monsters' in the bedroom

Setting up a solid bedroom routine, giving your child a special object for sleep and making sure they're in their own bed at night won't automatically banish those 'monsters' from the room.

Whether children are scared by actual monsters or subtler fears, never scold them or tell them they are just being a baby. It's always better to **try to understand** why they may be feeling insecure.

The key to night-time fears is to work out **how frightened children actually are**. They tend to say they are more frightened than is really the case. Sometimes they are not frightened at all, but say they are because they've learned this will always make you come to them.

If your child says they are afraid but there are no real signs of panic, then it is time to be firm. Stick to the bedtime routine you've established. Simply reassure them firmly and matter-of-factly that they are safe, put them to bed with the usual story or quiet talk, then leave. Do not return repeatedly. They will be less fearful in the long run if you show them you can take care of them without giving in to their worries.

However, there are times when **children *do* become extremely frightened at night**, panicked and irrational. Their emotional conflicts have got out of hand. Being firm simply will not work, and in fact will just make matters worse.

If they begin to have difficulty going to sleep because they are worried or fearful at bedtime, it is crucial to talk it over with them during the day. Empathy, reassurance and support are the **catalysts for change** here. It's important not to make any substantial changes to their bedtime routine. Physically and mentally reassure them, but try to stay on their normal schedule.

If their fears concern *literal* monsters, it may be helpful before bed to show them that any shadows in the wardrobe are in fact not monsters at all. It *isn't* useful to do extended searches of the room, or rearrange the furniture during the night. While the monsters are not real, your child's urges and worries are. They don't understand that it is these feelings, rather than monsters, that are making them anxious.

Help them **use their imagination** to explain their feelings: find something that they can believe is the *cause* of their fears and monsters. They need to know that nothing bad will happen if they wet or soil the bed, have a temper tantrum or feel anger towards their siblings.

If they have their own room and seem afraid to be in it alone at night, it may be useful to **spend time with them there during the day**, reading, talking or playing games. Gradually, you can encourage them to spend more time in their room without you, first during the day and then at night-time, so as to raise their comfort levels.

At first you should be more lenient with them when they go to bed. Sit with them if necessary. But as the intensity of their fear decreases, you will have to be firmer to re-establish normal routines, and prevent any temporary adjustments from becoming permanent so they are still able to fall asleep alone.

It is your calmness, firmness and loving reassurance that will remove the monsters from the room. Whatever their age, and whatever type of 'monster' they're afraid of, the best way to reassure them is to tell them that **you are in complete control**, and that you will protect them and keep them safe. If you can convince them of this, they will be able to relax.

If your child's fear is recent, even if it seems pronounced, with your support it will likely disappear **within a few weeks**. If they are still extremely fearful and show no signs of improvement after four weeks, and being firm just leads to further crying, panic and even hysteria, then you should seek **outside help**.

Many factors, from their age and stage of development to particular life circumstances, can contribute to such intense fears. The key here is you do not have to deal with them alone, and seeking help is OK. Experts in this area can help with any deeper issues that may underlie the anxiety, fear and emotional upset that give rise to disturbed sleep not just for the child but also for everyone else in the family.

Your calmness, firmness and loving reassurance will remove the monsters from your child's room.

PROBLEM 2:
WAKING DURING
THE NIGHT

As we saw in **Part 2**, brief awakenings at night are a normal part of sleep, for both children and adults. Our transitions between non-REM and REM sleep will be marked by short arousals, with movements such as adjusting the covers and looking around us, before we return to sleep. During these arousals we change body positions, which is important to our physical wellbeing, and briefly check our environment to make sure everything is as it should be.

But, as we saw with adults, if anything seems strange when children wake briefly, or not the same as it was when they went to sleep – if the light level has changed, for instance, and it's now **completely dark** – they can become more fully aroused. This is a particular problem for children when they have not learned to **build good associations** for sleep.

Other things can wake them too, such as **nightmares**, or – even more disturbing for those around them – conditions such as **sleep talking**, **sleepwalking** and **sleep terrors**. But never fear: even if they suffer from such disturbances as these, **nearly all children are potentially** *excellent sleepers* with just a little intervention.

Let's look at the surprisingly straightforward solutions to these problems.

Building good associations for *excellent sleep*

Most parents and carers don't realise that what they see as abnormal wakings during the night are actually quite normal. It is what they do to try to *fix* these 'abnormal' wakings – like going in to help their child go back to sleep – that is causing the disturbance.

We saw in the previous chapter that all children learn to associate certain **rituals**, **objects** and **conditions** with falling asleep. For most children this means a special time with their parent or carer, perhaps involving play or a story, and maybe being rocked to sleep; holding a favourite stuffed animal or special blanket; and being in a particular room, lying in a certain bed or cot. When they wake at night between sleep cycles in the normal way, and such conditions are still present, they return to sleep quickly.

However, if the conditions under which a child fell asleep have changed when they wake normally during the night, they will be **unable to fall straight back to sleep**. They will sense something is wrong, because **the conditions they have learned to associate with falling asleep**, like rocking and rubbing, **are no longer present**.

The brain, even in these early stages of development, has a strong sense of **association**, and the absence of familiar conditions will be seen as an early warning sign of danger. The child will wake up more fully and seek help by crying. Rather than brief, their arousal will be prolonged, because they have not learned how to return to sleep on their own. Hence, the problem is not one of abnormal waking, but one of **difficulty in falling back to sleep**.

As adults, we tend to take our associations with falling asleep for granted. But they are actually very important to us. We all learn to fall asleep under a certain group of conditions. We go to sleep on one side of the bed; we like certain pillows and blankets; before sleep we listen to music, or read another chapter of our book. If the routine varies, sometimes we will experience difficulty falling asleep.

What would happen if you woke up normally during the night to discover your pillow gone? Rather than simply returning to sleep, you would wake more completely and begin to look for it.

It might simply have fallen on the floor, in which case you would pick it up and probably get back to sleep quickly. But what if it were really gone? What if a very poor prank were pulled on you while you slept? You certainly *wouldn't* go straight back to sleep. It's highly likely you'd turn on the light, get out of bed and begin searching for your pillow. You might even get angry and frustrated – just like a child who wakes to changed conditions.

Babies and younger children

When a child is still in a bassinet or crib, sorting out improper sleep associations is fairly straightforward, and the improvement will be very rapid. For a baby, marked improvement should occur **within a few days**, and certainly **within a week or two**. What you need to do is teach them a new group of sleep associations. While you are doing this you are going to need patience, understanding and most importantly consistency, until they adapt to the new pattern. There will be some crying, but it should be at a minimum.

To understand this, I want you to think about the pillow example again. If it became necessary for you to sleep without a pillow (due to neck issues, for instance), you would find it difficult to begin with. You would probably be uncomfortable at bedtime and take a long time to get yourself into a good position for sleep. You would probably curse your bad neck, even though you understood the importance of sleeping without a pillow. You would finally drift off, but find it difficult to fall back to sleep after night-time arousals.

The only way you could learn to fall asleep without a pillow would be to **practise** doing it. Each time you fell asleep without a pillow it would become easier, until at last it would begin to feel OK. At this point, prolonged night-time waking would also diminish.

You cannot learn how to fall asleep without a pillow if you go to sleep with a pillow every night but have someone take it away after you are sleeping soundly. You need to be without a pillow each and every time you fall asleep. To break your child's unhelpful sleep associations, they will need to **learn to fall asleep *without* the things that will not be there if they wake during the night**. For a child to learn to fall asleep without being nursed, rocked or held, without radio or TV, or without a pacifier, **none of these sleep helpers should be present at any of the times they go to sleep**. Not at bedtime, nap time or times when they wake up through the night.

Breaking the association of **nursing** with falling asleep is not necessary to wean your child. It is only necessary to dissociate the two. Instead of nursing at bedtime, you could nurse earlier in the evening. During the day, you could nurse earlier instead of at nap time. If they start to fall asleep while feeding, stop and place them into their cot and let them fall asleep in that setting.

Excessive feeding can be problematic. If they are taking a lot of fluid at night, from you or the bottle, their sleep may be disturbed in several ways other than the effects of the sleep associations. However, suddenly stopping the feeding at night would be difficult on the child and difficult for you. It would be better to gradually reduce the number and frequency of feeds.

If they prefer a **pacifier** only when going to sleep, then once they learn to fall asleep without it, they will no longer use it at all. But if they have it in their mouth most of the day, then it is going to be very much more difficult to remove it when night time comes. You could firstly decrease the amount of pacifier time during the day, and be there to give them extra attention and provide diversions to make the adjustment easier. You may have to listen to a little crying as they learn to be comfortable without the pacifier, just as when they're learning new associations for night time.

The key is to decide on certain periods of the day when they should not use the pacifier. Increase these periods gradually. Once they are using the pacifier mainly when wanting to sleep, you can eliminate it completely and begin the progressive conditioning already discussed. By that point they will be quite used to being without a pacifier when awake, and will only have to learn how to sleep without it.

*

This **progressive conditioning** approach works very well with children, but you do need to ensure that the changes are **gradual**. Children learning new rules will not understand them at first. They need to know you are nearby and ready to take care of them. They can only learn this through experience.

If you let them cry alone each night and do not return at all until morning, they will still learn that you always come back eventually and that you are not really abandoning them, but the lesson will be unnecessarily difficult. If you wait a short period of time before going to them, then increase the waiting time progressively, the lesson will be much easier.

Initially they will be unhappy as they try to learn to fall asleep in this new way, but they will soon find out that you are still around and ready to respond, and then there will be much less uncertainty. They will begin to realise what you have planned. They will start expecting you to gradually increase the waiting time.

Using this progressive technique, you are helping them to *minimise* crying, while the cold-turkey technique will only lead to *maximum* crying. If you stick to the old method of comforting them whenever they cry during the night, things will not improve no matter how much crying there is.

When you *do* go to them, **stay with them for a short time only**. Eventually they will learn it is no longer worth the twenty minutes of crying just to have you come in briefly. Do not sit or lie on their bed, and always make sure they fall asleep when you are **out of the room**. Remember, better sleep, and eventually *excellent sleep*, come only when they learn how to *fall* asleep, and *return* to sleep, alone.

If they do wake at night, they know you will come, but there will be very little to gain with no holding, rocking and so on. If you make the night-time waking **pleasurable** – holding them, rocking them, playing with them – it will nourish their brain's pleasure centres and they will be motivated to continue waking at night. Even if you scold or punish them when you go to them, waking up may still be rewarded by the attention they get.

This is especially so if they get very little attention during the day, and particularly if they spend too little time with you alone. If this is the case, try to set aside **special times** for them during the day. When they feel less needy, they are less likely to demand attention at night. If providing extra time is not possible, or they seem needy regardless of the extra time, then it may be helpful to talk with a counsellor to dig more deeply into the sleep issue.

Older children

For older children, intervention sometimes has to proceed a bit more slowly, but should be just as successful. The child must still learn to fall asleep with the same set of conditions that will be present at the times of normal wakings through the night – the most important being that **they must be alone in bed**.

If they are used to having you in bed with them when they fall asleep, you may be able to break the association in a number of ways. If they're old enough, you could simply explain to them that you can no longer lie down with them while they fall asleep. Just make sure you compensate with **a pleasant and appropriate bedtime ritual**.

When you finish telling them a story, or whatever it might be, tuck them in then leave the room, but keep the door open. Some children will **call out or cry**; others will **get out of bed**. If they simply **call out or cry**, then progressively increase the amount of time between your brief responses to them. The second night, wait longer before your first response, wait longer still on the third night, and so on.

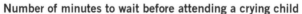

Number of minutes to wait before attending a crying child

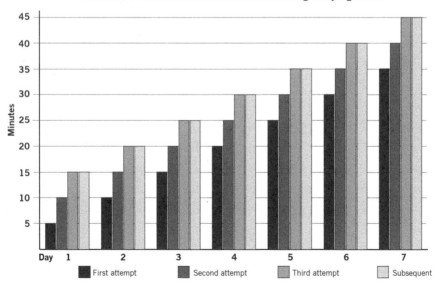

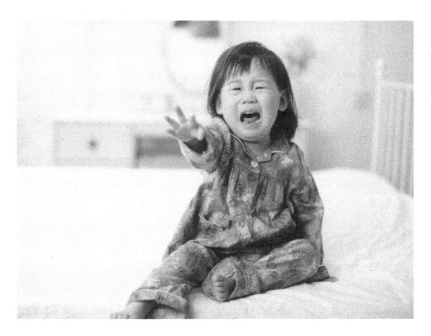

Use the graph on the previous page as a guide to the number of minutes you should wait before going to a crying child. As you can see, you should be able to increase the waiting time quite dramatically in as little as a week.

When you go in, **spend only two to three minutes with your child**. The idea is to briefly reassure them; you should not aim to stop them crying or help them fall asleep at this stage, as **your overall goal is for them to fall asleep on their own** without needing to be comforted or given a pacifier.

If you get to the maximum number of minutes for the night, continue leaving for that amount of time until the child finally falls asleep when you are out of the room. If they wake up during the night, start again at the minimum waiting time and work up to the maximum as per the table.

Continue this routine after any waking until morning – usually any time between 5.30 and 7.30am, as suits your routine.

When it comes to **naps**, use the same schedule, but if your child has not fallen asleep after one hour, or if they wake again and start crying vigorously after getting some sleep, end that naptime period.

Be sure to follow your schedule carefully and **keep a record** so you can monitor progress. It is highly likely that by the seventh day your child will be sleeping very well. But if further work is necessary, just continue to add five minutes to each time on successive days.

*

If your child **gets out of bed**, you will require a different tactic. When you are certain they are out of the bed, go into the room, put them back into bed and tell them to stay in bed or **you will have to close the door**. Most children are very uncomfortable sleeping in totally enclosed spaces, as it only reinforces their sense of separation from you. (As we'll see on pages 171 to 172, they also get uncomfortable in total darkness.)

If they get out of bed *again*, put them back to bed and close the door for **about a minute**. **Don't lock the door**, but hold it closed if they try to open it. Locking a child in a room is very scary for them and will not help the new learning process.

You want to demonstrate that the issue of whether the door is open or shut is **under their control**. If they stay in bed, the door stays open; if they get out of bed, the door stays closed. Use of a **gate** is also OK, as long as they are unable to open it and you are out of view when it is closed.

Talking to your child in a reassuring manner through a closed door, or from another room using a gate, will let them know you are still nearby. Tell them that if they get back into bed you will be able to reopen the door after the minute is up.

If they still don't get back into bed, go in, put them down, close the door and this time wait **two minutes**. If this pattern continues, increase the time you keep the door closed to **three minutes**, and the next time to **five minutes**. Five minutes should be the maximum for the first night.

When your child finally *does* stay in bed or goes back to bed on their own, open the door after the time is up, give them a few words of encouragement and leave without going into the room.

If they start getting out of bed later, after night-time wakings, make sure to follow the same routine used at bedtime, starting again at one minute.

On the **second night**, at bedtime or after night-time wakings, start at **two minutes**. Increase the time each subsequent night.

You may want to use the following chart as a guide to how many minutes to keep the door closed at each stage.

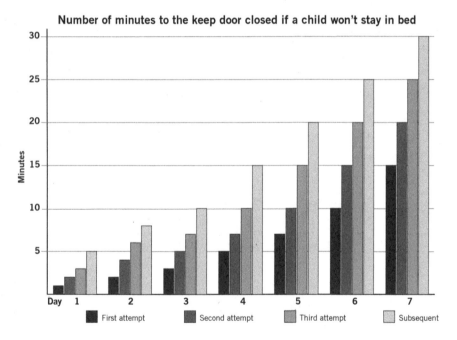

Number of minutes to the keep door closed if a child won't stay in bed

Nap times will also have to be controlled with the door-closing technique, but if your child has not fallen asleep after one hour, or if they are awake again after a period of sleep, make that the end of the nap for the day.

Simple door-closing is a much more controlled pattern of enforcement than trying to hold them in bed, or getting frustrated and spanking them. Children should never be threatened or spanked when they won't stay in bed; it will only make things worse. You need them to know that you want to help them learn the new sleep routine with **support, not punishment**.

This form of progressive conditioning will not be easy, because the child's brain has patterns that are being upset, and they will need time to establish new patterns. Children will vary in how much pushback their brain will exert. Some will learn quickly that they would rather stay in bed and have the door open than get out of bed and have the door closed even briefly. Others will continue getting out of bed a number of times, being willing to accept longer periods of door closure before giving in.

This brain change will likely take longer than with a child confined to a crib, but if you persevere, their brain will accept the new pattern. Things will be much better **within a week, two at the very most**.

Consistency is the important element here. If you are lenient sometimes and firm at other times, they will always be waiting for you to give in.

*

When your child reaches **three or so**, it may also help to use a **reward system** to help the initial phase of brain relearning happen much faster. Adopt this system either **before** or **during** the door-closing technique. Try rewards such as stickers and occasionally larger prizes for going to sleep without getting out of bed. This will motivate them to try to go to sleep without you in the room, and will help them feel that you and they are working together to improve the situation.

Remember, when the novelty of rewards begins to wear off, the demands around bedtime may escalate once again. When this happens, you will have to be especially careful not to give in, or the child's brain will return to its old patterns very quickly.

*

If all of this is too much for them to process in one or two weeks, you will need to move at **a more gradual pace**. They may then have to relearn each step along the way.

Tell them that you cannot be in bed with them when they fall asleep, but instead of leaving the room, **sit on a chair near their bed** until they fall asleep. If they try to get out of bed, then begin the door-closing routine. When you return, make sure it is to the same chair. They will learn that, through their own behaviour, they control whether you are in the room near them, or out of the room with the door (or gate) closed. If they can't have you in bed with them, they will quickly learn that it is better to have you nearby than outside the door.

Once they have learned to fall asleep – or to get back to sleep after waking – alone in their bed but with you still in the room, you have helped them through a major part of the process.

You can then move forward in one- to two-week intervals. You will need to move your chair progressively further away from their bed until you are just outside their bedroom door or gate. In the end you should be able to leave the bedtime area completely after saying goodnight. Each step should be reinforced with the door-closing technique as required.

As with the quicker approach, many variations are possible, and there may be difficulties at each step. Getting out of their bed will be the hardest step; the second hardest will be taking yourself right out of the room.

If your child appears particularly anxious, then I highly recommend this gradual approach. But the less protracted method works the best, because the new sleep pattern is achieved much more quickly, meaning there is only *one* difficult period of relearning. With the gradual approach, the time it takes them to fall asleep tends to be longer, since they know that you will leave once they fall asleep, and so they may begin to fight sleep, rousing themselves each time they enter a drowsy state.

*

Whichever method you use, when your child has learned how to fall asleep on their own, it is no longer a matter of teaching them how to do it, but simply of reinforcing the new rules. If they relapse into the old pattern, then being firm and, if necessary, restarting the door-closing routine, will ensure that they return to the desired sleep pattern very quickly.

It's dark in here

Just as most children prefer having the door left open at night, they also feel uncomfortable when left in total darkness. There is no advantage in trying to train them to sleep completely in the dark.

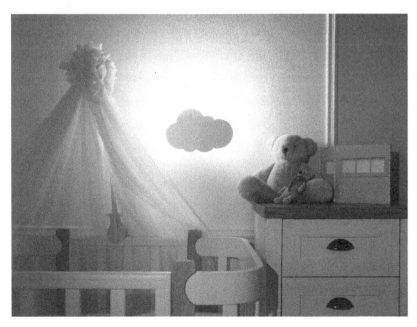

It's very helpful for the bedroom to be **dimly lit** by anything like a soft light, a hall light, or even an outside light, so that when they wake up during the night, particularly after a dream, they can reorient themselves within the room, get their sense of reality back and put any dreams they were having into proper perspective.

If they have anxieties at bedtime or after night-time wakings, they may get some reassurance from being able to see around their room. As we've seen, some children have fears of **shadows** and **monsters under the bed**. In this case, try altering the lighting pattern in the room, and once you find one that works, stick with it. Just like pretending to search for the monsters or rearranging furniture, turning lights on and off or moving them around the room each night will do little to change their fears.

Once again, **bedtime associations** are important here. If they fall asleep with a particular light on at bedtime, but become frightened on waking during the night after you have turned the light off, then you should leave the light on all night.

Nightmares

We all, including children now and then, have nightmares. However, for children they are not the common cause of frequent night-time disturbances. As we're about to learn, what we might consider frequent nightmares are really **sleep terrors**, or similar partial wakings.

When children *do* wake up frightened from a scary dream, they should not have to stay alone. But you certainly want to avoid having to stay with them on a regular or nightly basis.

One approach to avoiding this would be to discuss the dream matter-of-factly, either at the time or in the morning. This will help them reorient themselves and realise there is no real danger.

Sleep terrors, talks and walks

A baby who wakes crying ... a toddler who thrashes bizarrely ... a young child who talks in their sleep ... an older child who sleepwalks then wakes frightened as if from a bad dream ... a pre-adolescent who runs and thrashes frantically at night ... and an adolescent who runs around widely in terror and sometimes even injures themselves.

What do they have in common? They all have a similar underlying sleep issue, which is **an incomplete waking from non-dreaming sleep**. The detailed characteristics and the significance of these arousals vary, depending on age and physiological and emotional factors.

Sleep talking and walking have always been the most curious of sleep disturbances and may be regarded as disorders when severe. They are well known and worrisome to parents. **Sleep terrors** are far more dramatic, and frightening to most families who have to experience them first-hand.

Less intense but lengthier periods of **confused thrashing** can be just as disturbing for parents. They are almost universally misinterpreted as bad dreams that can be stopped by waking the child up, or as epileptic seizures that will require specialist attention.

Because these disorders are not commonly discussed among adults or children, many view these behaviours as abnormal. But in fact they are fairly common and – you'll be pleased to hear – are generally outgrown over time.

Sleepwalking

At some stage of the night, usually one to four hours after falling asleep, a child may start **moaning, speaking unintelligibly and moving restlessly** for a few minutes. They may lift their head, sit up briefly, grind their teeth and look about confusedly before falling back to sleep. Their behaviour may appear odd; they may be distressed, confused, disoriented and unable to recognise where they are. If the episode becomes particularly intense, they can move about the bed as if looking for something, and in some cases may even **move out of the bed and start walking around**.

At least 15 per cent of children have had at least one sleepwalking episode. It may look the same at any age, but with older children the level of agitation can increase.

Though the child appears to be awake, since their eyes are open, they can't manage any complex actions requiring higher, frontal-lobe levels of mental functioning like memory recall or reading. They in fact have very little awareness of what is going on around them. They won't recognise you, but more often than not will still come towards you, at which point they will stare *through* you, not at you. This is particularly true if they are beyond the toddler phase.

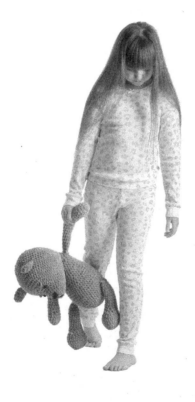

Disconcertingly, they can also **walk down stairs** and sometimes, if able, will **leave the house**. During this activity they will be calm and will respond with simple, usually one-word answers. If told to go back to bed, they may do so, or they may let you take them back, often with a bathroom stop on the way. (Unfortunately, boys are more likely to go to the toilet somewhere *other* than the toilet because of confusion. Wardrobes, bins and shoes are the most likely recipients.)

Sometimes these behaviours are **far less calm and much louder**. The child may jump out of bed and run around the house, appearing quite agitated and confused, as if they are trying to get away from something. Expressions of anger or apprehension are common. They may feel along the bedroom walls, even hitting furniture, people and surfaces, so that falling and injuring themselves becomes a distinct possibility. While all of this may be over in a minute, they will remain confused for at least two or three minutes afterwards.

In **less than forty minutes – usually twenty at most –** the episode will end fairly suddenly, and you can learn to recognise this. There will be a general relaxation, including stretching and yawning, and they will go back to their bed quite quickly.

Once back in bed, younger children will simply go back to sleep without ever really waking up. Older children may wake up fully, either spontaneously or in response to your actions. They will have no memory of the event, and will seem calm and unworried – probably the opposite of what *you* are feeling. If they do seem to be upset, it will be because they are embarrassed that they found themselves in some unexpected place with people staring at them.

Sleep terrors

Very young children are extremely unlikely to demonstrate agitated sleepwalking, but their **intense arousals** can still

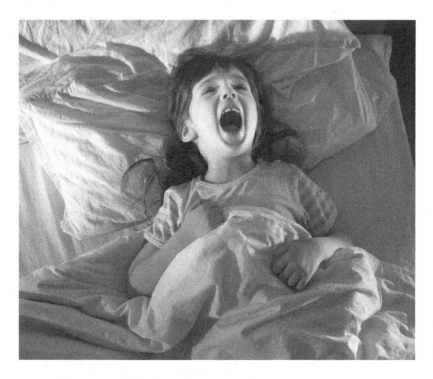

seem bizarre and frightening to us. These occurrences are known as **sleep terrors** or **night terrors**, even though the child does not look frightened during the episode, or in any pain.

A partial waking up, with lots of crying and little ability to calm down, can occur **as early as six months of age**. This generally doesn't seem strange to us, because the tossing and turning are not severe, and we have a tendency to expect these very young ones to have periods of uncontrolled crying. You may simply assume the child has had a bad dream, an assumption that's easy to make when it's impossible to ask them. However, it's important that you learn to recognise this behaviour in infants and toddlers, because it's very different from the night wakings we've discussed so far, which have been to do with habits and associations.

These arousals affect children of all ages, but happen most frequently in adolescents (aged thirteen to eighteen), and to a slightly lesser extent pre-adolescents (aged nine to twelve).

Typically a sleep terror can start very suddenly. The child may wake up and go through a long period of moaning, then suddenly start crying, or let out a horrible scream and sit rigidly upright in bed.

They may toss and turn in bed with their eyes bulging and a strange look on their face, as if they are terrified, agitated and upset. They may sweat and if you touch their chest you may feel their heart pounding. They may often yell about being attacked or trapped, or falling.

Tossing and turning is uncommon as children get older, but more distinct sleep terrors may become apparent. For older children these episodes can be much shorter than the tossing and turning of younger children, and often end in less than five minutes. When they wake, usually briefly, they go back to sleep quickly. Again, when they are fully awake they will have no memory of anything, except occasionally of some of the words that were used during the event. They cannot describe the event in any detail that would suggest it was actually a dream.

The strange facial expression, together with the tossing and turning and lack of response to you, can create an eerie effect. All of this will be quite foreign and strange to you in terms of their day behaviours, and you'll probably assume they are having a bad dream.

This tossing and turning, sobbing and moaning will generally last **from ten to forty minutes, though sometimes as long as sixty**. After that they'll simply yawn, stretch and lie back down. Interestingly, if they are sitting during this stage, they will not let you help them lie down or tuck them in. If they do wake up fully they will be calm and just go back to sleep. If you try to keep them awake, usually because you want to be sure they are OK, they may stay awake for a few more minutes but will soon be asleep without any memory of the night's events.

So what exactly is happening?

Sleep terrors, sleepwalking, sleep talking and thrashing in bed are not stimulated by dreams. We know that these episodes do not happen during the dream stage, because the near-paralysis that occurs during REM sleep (which we read about on pages 12 and 40) effectively prevents this from happening. We cannot sit up, thrash about, walk, run or even scream. However, during non-REM sleep we *can* move, and usually do, at least during the transitions between sleep cycles.

The disorders we've been discussing all occur during **partial waking from Stage 4 non-REM sleep**. They happen when both the sleeping and waking patterns are working together, indicating that the child is simultaneously awake and asleep.

To understand this better, let's look at children's sleep cycles in more detail.

As we saw in **WHAT HAPPENS WHEN CHILDREN SLEEP** (pages 132 to 137), from the age of three months, children go straight into non-REM sleep, reaching **Stage 4** after about ten minutes. They will remain in Stage 4 for about an hour, then this period will end suddenly with a brief arousal. This partial waking may last for only a few seconds or up to several minutes. Occasionally a child may briefly wake up fully, and sometimes Stage 4 will merge almost imperceptibly with REM sleep with no arousal.

After a short REM episode, or an attempt to form REM sleep, they will return to another cycle of non-REM sleep. In young children, the descent back into Stage 4 for the second sleep cycle will be quite rapid, but not as fast as the first. After forty to fifty minutes there will be another arousal.

Sleep terrors, talks and walks occur most often during these arousals at the end of the **first** or **second sleep cycle, between one and four hours** after sleep begins.

Stage 4 sleep is an extremely deep sleep, and waking a child can be almost impossible, even with vigorous shaking. During this stage we can carry a sleeping child from the car and put them into their pyjamas and then bed with no arousal. Even if we wake a child to go to the toilet during Stage 4, they remain in a semi-awake state and will have no recollection of the arousal in the morning. The arousal is only partial in this situation. And it's very similar to what happens during the partial arousals between sleep cycles.

There is **a spectrum of behaviours** that may occur during these arousal periods. In sleep laboratory conditions, a child being monitored will show nothing to indicate that a change in their sleep state is about to occur. Then they will move suddenly and without warning. Their brain waves will change abruptly, showing a mixture of patterns from deep sleep, light sleep, drowsiness and even waking. They may rub their face, chew, turn over, cry a little or speak unintelligibly. They may even open their eyes for a moment with a blank stare or sit up briefly before falling back into a deeper sleep and starting the next sleep cycle.

Mild behaviours like these are quite common. Other behaviours that occur during these partial wakings – sleepwalking, sleep terrors, confused thrashing and sometimes bedwetting – are *not* so common. For some children, this transition between sleep states does not happen quickly or smoothly, and they proceed to walk, scream or even run around. This is almost always related to the depth of the child's Stage 4 sleep, as well as their level of development.

Sometimes the triggers are **external**, such as the wakings referred to above, or when you make noises in or outside their room, or a movement such as pulling their blanket a little higher. These disturbances are most likely to trigger a partial awakening if they happen near the end of Stage 4 sleep. The sound of something quite loud about an hour after going to sleep can trigger sleep terrors in some children. Even children who have never been sleepwalkers can become so if you make them stand up around this time.

It is very likely that the stimuli triggering these arousals at the end of the first or second sleep cycle are too small to fully break the ongoing deep sleep state. Because of this, the child can be left in a variable state where they are **half asleep and half awake**.

So how does this feel for them? Imagine that, after an hour of sleep, you heard an alarm, gunfire or a very loud scream. You would wake up instantly but your head would feel 'woolly', like it was filled with cobwebs, as you tried to figure out what was happening. You would probably notice your heart racing. You would feel scared and compelled to do something, yet you would still find it took several seconds or even longer to act.

That period of a few seconds during which you feel afraid but not yet fully alert is just like what children experience during sleepwalking, talking and terrors, even though they don't remember it afterwards.

*

In most cases children **outgrow** sleep terrors by **six years old**, with their most common occurrences being around the age of three or four. Up to the age of six, these episodes are rarely caused by physical or emotional problems, but are generally part of **normal maturing**. There are other possible causes too, including **hormonal** and other **biological changes**. Many children have **close relatives** with a history of similar events. In very young children this may explain the occurrence of night-time arousals completely.

Occasionally, though, **psychological factors** may be involved. If there is significant stress at home, or if the episodes began after a specific period of upset, it may be necessary to seek professional advice.

*

As our children move through **middle childhood** (six to twelve) and **adolescence** (thirteen to eighteen), these night-time events may show many different characteristics and levels of intensity, as well as many causes. In older children they are less likely to be developmental. Stage 4 non-REM sleep is very deep in young children, but deeper in older children and extremely deep in adults. So older children should be able to make the transition from Stage 4 to the next sleep cycle smoothly. Any extreme response to night-time arousals is more likely to result from **emotional factors**, particularly if the episodes become more frequent.

There is no specific age below which all such arousals are developmental and above which they are emotional. But if the child is older than six and night-time wakings persist, or appear for the first time, there is likely to be a psychological component. Just as for children under six, a **family history** of the disorder could explain why some older children develop these sleeping problems.

It is important to consider **how often** older children experience these extreme night-time arousals, and the context in which they occur. Sleepwalking or similar events, and the possible underlying psychological issues, are of little consequence if such episodes occur only once a year.

For **frequent** sleep terrors or sleepwalking to occur after the age of six or seven, the child needs **both a biological and an emotional predisposition**. Not only the frequency but also the intensity of the occurrences will be determined by this combination of inherited and psychological traits.

The data shows that the emotional problems children experience are not necessarily major ones. They are usually to do with how the child deals with their feelings. Typically, a well-behaved child will **find it difficult to outwardly express**

any feelings they consider negative, such as anger, hate, guilt and jealousy.

Older children often find themselves in situations where they feel like the things happening to them are outside their control, such as when they move house or change schools. But it is following losses such as parental separation or divorce or a death in the family that psychological factors generally emerge. Even if the family is intact, there may an absence of love or warmth. Parents who are rigid and demanding and have high expectations regarding behaviour, school performance and even sporting success can leave their child angry about their circumstances but unable to express that anger outwardly.

Instead, they **remain on guard**, believing that if they express their feelings it may only lead to further deterioration and unpleasantness. They may already blame themselves for any family problems that have occurred. They view emotion as the enemy, something to be kept in check. They will avoid behaviour that could lead to displeasure and will often pretend to be coping well by being well behaved and

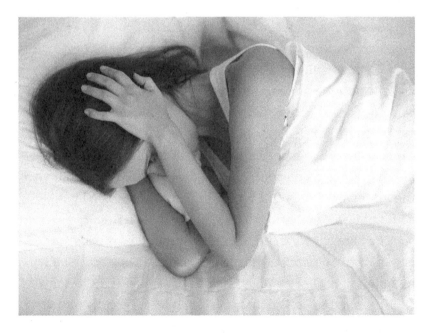

pleasant – perhaps overly so. Occasionally they will show their anger in passive ways that feel safe.

They tend to use an enormous amount of energy during the day guarding their emotions, but at night when sleep they are relaxed and their defences are down. During a partial arousal after the first or second sleep cycle, they find themselves confused and out of control. Before they know what is happening, a fearful response is generated by their autonomic nervous system. It doesn't require complex thought processes for this fear to be expressed in the form of sleep terrors and similar episodes.

An older child's arousals may be **different on different nights**, or at **different stages of their development**. Often they will show a progression from quiet arousals to major sleep terrors, usually because of changes in life stresses and the manner in which they are dealt with. Daily changes, and their night-time consequences, may be **subtle and difficult to recognise**. Night-time arousals usually wax and wane over weeks and months without any noticeable daytime changes. Hence, it is not easy to predict when a child will have night-time episodes based on awareness of the daytime stresses they are currently facing.

It may be the case that night-time episodes **decrease** when they start to misbehave, or become temperamental or uncooperative. When they allow themselves to express their feelings during the day, however inappropriately, they will have less need to guard against these feelings and are more likely to sleep without interruption.

It is very rare that **medical problems** underlie these arousals in older children, though occasionally they are the result of illness such as fever. If it is one of these rare occasions, the child will wake up at times outside the usual Stage 4 waking. They will have more general sleep disruption, and only some of the arousals will involve sleepwalking or sleep terrors.

Very rarely, **night-time epileptic seizures** can mimic sudden partial wakings. If the arousals occur nearer morning rather than closer to bedtime, and the child wakes fully at the start and realises that something is about to occur, or if they have a good memory of the entire event, or of its beginning, then you may be dealing with epilepsy and will need to seek expert help. If the episodes are always exactly the same, and there is marked body stiffening with one arm extended and the head turned to the side, or there is prominent repetitive body jerking, you should also seek expert professional help.

*

So **which comes first? The terror or the arousal?** There is much debate among researchers in this area. Some believe the terror comes first and causes a sudden arousal, while others think arousal comes first, followed by the physiological responses associated with fear.

This distinction is most important for children above six years of age, when – as we've seen – emotional factors become more relevant. Some feel that the arousal is **triggered by frightening thoughts or images** that suddenly enter into the child's consciousness during the deep sleep state, when their emotional defences are down. These scary thoughts cause them to scream and have a partial waking.

However, this does not explain why a sleep terror can be triggered by noise, and it does not explain why sleep terrors tend to occur at the end of the first and second sleep cycle, rather than interrupting an ongoing sleep stage.

The alternative view is that **the arousal comes first**, caused by an underlying sleep problem or even by sound. Increased heart rate, sweating and other bodily changes associated with fear occur simply as part of this sudden arousal from Stage 4 sleep. Thus, these children wake partially and find themselves in a state of agitation, to which they respond by crying out, running all over the place, or muttering gibberish.

The idea that arousal comes first appears to be the best explanation as to why children don't have any clear memories of the event afterwards, and why, as the event ends and their heart rate and other bodily functions return to normal, they experience no lingering fears.

The **actual trigger** is in all likelihood only **the normal mechanisms that control the end of one sleep cycle and the start of another**: a component of the biorhythms controlling our internal clock. This is why the events occur when we would normally expect the first or second sleep cycle to end.

This does not mean that **emotional factors** are not relevant, it's just that the emotional stress acts **indirectly**. Emotional factors do not *trigger* the arousals, but they may well affect how the child responds. (This is different from a **nightmare**, in which the stressful daytime event may appear in the dream in a symbolic form, which in turn would generate enough anxiety to wake them up. After a nightmare they will still feel fearful and generally will be able to remember what happened.)

What can I do to help them?

We can all feel empathy towards a child who wakes up at night frightened and distressed, and who can be made to feel better with a little comforting. But when you attempt to help your child yet are pushed aside, you can feel **angry**, particularly if you don't understand what's happening to them. Watching them thrash wildly about in the bed for what seems an eternity can be **frightening**.

It's particularly important that you try not to overreact during these periods of partial arousal. Suspend thoughts of 'They are possessed', so that you can maintain your own psychological balance. No amount of stimulation can shorten one of these episodes – at least not a major one. The event will continue to run its course, and usually will only be intensified if you try to **hold or restrain them**. There is very little chance they will respond to you. They will seem to perceive your actions as a threat instead of a help, perhaps because they feel you closing in on them but they don't recognise you. They will reject any comforting behaviour from you and will most likely **push you away**. You should simply try to watch the episode proceed, conscious that nothing serious is happening. Whatever is going on, the key is just to **wait**.

It is important not to **wake** them after one of these events, and most certainly not to **question** them, either at the time or when they wake in the morning. They can become quite angry when asked over and over about the content of their 'dream', because they are concerned about their loss of control during the night. Interrogating them just leads to escalation of bedtime worries, and even more arousal events in the future. It only makes sense to tell them about their arousal episodes if they ask, or if they are old enough to make their own decisions about seeking further help in the form of expert advice.

In the case of **sleepwalking**, you can lead a calm sleepwalker back to bed, but if they become agitated you will want to wait until they calm down again. Obviously **safety** is a priority, and you will need to deal with obstacles on the floor and entry points to stairs. If the child is older, you will need to take extra precautions so they do not leave the house.

If possible, you should allow even full **sleep terrors** to run their course. Obviously there will be times when you will need to intervene, and in these circumstances you will need to do so as calmly and gently as possible. If the episodes are unusually frequent, intense or even dangerous, you may need to seek **expert advice**.

*

Infants and toddlers who have **occasional** tossing, turning and thrashing do not need your help. They need you to keep your distance and let the episode run its course, and they will eventually return to sleep.

Younger children up to the age of six can be helped by ensuring **adequate amounts of sleep at night**. Most of us expect an overtired child to sleep better, but usually this is not the case. They are more likely to suffer sleep terrors or simply sleepwalk. This happens because a sleep-deprived child has a greater need for deep sleep, which may prevent the deep sleep system from giving way at the end of the first or second sleep cycle, leading to a state of partially waking up.

You also need to ensure your younger child has a **regular schedule**. If they are having these partial wakings, then try to make sure their bed and nap times are regular. (Read **FINDING THE BEST DAILY SCHEDULE** on pages 138 to 143 for some pointers.) If you do this, their biorhythms will become more stable and begin to work in harmony again.

While adequate sleep, normal schedules and keeping your distance are good for dealing with arousal problems in young children, they don't always provide the total answer. If your child is susceptible to these episodes, pay attention to their frequency and nature, and in particular any **stresses** you can identify that may be part of the overall picture.

Medications are generally a poor choice for younger children, as the side effects tend to outweigh the benefits. Medications may be necessary if there is potential for the child to injure themselves, but this is a low risk before late childhood and adolescence.

In some instances you may just have to **learn to live with the arousals**. With time, understanding what is happening should lead to greater acceptance of any inconvenience the night wakings cause.

*

For older children – from six years to adolescence – the solution is for them to **learn to go to sleep without being on guard**, so that night-time arousals can proceed normally. They need to understand that their feelings are not dangerous and that there is no need to guard against expressing them. You and they may need **professional help** to guide you through, as this is certainly no easy lesson to learn.

The need to seek counselling or other professional assistance is clear when the child appears to be suffering from a great deal of stress that may or may not include sleep disturbance issues. If your child is feeling stressed multiple times during the week, then it would be wise to seek help. If their night-time episodes are dangerous – leading them to walk to stairways, for example – then you urgently need help, or at least an initial evaluation. Counselling will help reduce the arousals, even if no stresses seem apparent in your child and they are able to communicate with you quite well.

This psychotherapy is needed to identify and treat psychological problems, not simply to cure the arousal events. Although stopping the arousals may be a prime goal, you cannot **judge the success** of the therapy simply by keeping track of the frequency or intensity of the arousal episodes.

It may be that improvement in sleep follows progress in therapy **very slowly**. It may take some time for your child to learn new ways of dealing with important feelings, so that they are able to go to bed without worrying about what may happen if they relax their emotional defences in sleep.

The following table summarises the issues and solutions we have looked at above.

What you observe	Age	What to do
Continuous crying and sobbing, perhaps with wild thrashing	Usually six months to six years, occasionally older	Go in and check the child is not injuring themselves. Let the episode run its course. Hold the child if they recognise you and want to be held, but don't force anything. In particular, do not shake or attempt to wake the child. Watch for the calm that signals the end of this behaviour. Only then should you help them lie down and perhaps put their bedcovers back over them. Let them go back to sleep. Resist trying to wake or talk to them about what might be wrong or what they were dreaming, and do not question them in the morning, as it will only make them feel strange and different.
Sleepwalking but relatively calm while doing so	Any age from when the child becomes mobile	Talk quietly and calmly to your child. They may follow your instructions and go back to bed by themselves. If they are not upset when you reach out and touch them, you should be able to guide them calmly back to bed. They may want to stop at the bathroom. It's best not to wake them, but if they wake spontaneously, try not to be negative or critical. Again, don't mention it in the morning unless asked.
Sleepwalking and relatively agitated while doing so	Middle childhood through adolescence	Keep your distance. Only hold or restrain the child if they are in danger, as it will increase the intensity and duration of the episode. When they calm down, treat as for calm sleepwalking.
Sleep terrors: screaming, looking terrified and perhaps running about wildly	Late adolescence	Observe from a distance until the screaming subsides and to the child goes back to sleep. Only intervene if the child is in danger; do so with caution. Do not wake the child or quiz them about what is happening, as it will only embarrass them.

PROBLEM 3: CHILDREN'S BIOLOGICAL CLOCKS

The key to dealing with childhood sleep problems, and most importantly setting the parameters for *excellent sleep*, is understanding the circadian cycles that underlie children's sleep patterns.

As we learned in **Part 2**, we humans run into difficulties when our sleeping hours are not in sync with the rhythms of our **biological clock**. Shift workers are particularly prone to sleep problems, and people who travel across time zones generally suffer sleep difficulties and a lack of wellbeing that we commonly call jet lag.

It's the same with children who have sleep disturbances caused by problems in their patterns of sleeping and waking. As we saw in **FINDING THE BEST DAILY SCHEDULE** (pages 138 to 143), the importance of maintaining **consistent schedules** for our children is so very important throughout infancy, childhood and adolescence, although many parents do not seem to appreciate this. If children do not have reasonable consistency in their daily routines, their system does not know when they should be asleep or awake. If their circadian rhythm is disrupted, their usual pattern, which allows them to sleep for long periods at night and to nap during the day, will begin to evaporate.

It's asking for trouble to let your two- or three-year-old decide what time they should go to bed. It would usually be only when they were so sleepy they could no longer stay awake. Before long their schedule would become quite random and haphazard. They would fall asleep early one night and late the next. They might nap some days and not others. When they did nap, it might be in the morning, afternoon or early evening.

If this schedule were even further disrupted, mealtimes would also fluctuate all over the place. Breakfast might end up any time between seven and eleven in the morning. Lunch and dinner would also appear at odd times, or even be skipped altogether. This is major sleep problem territory, with all the behavioural problems that flow from it – subtle at first but ultimately highly detrimental.

As we saw in **Part 2**, our basic daily rhythms tend to run on a twenty-five hour cycle and we reset them to twenty-four hours through our daily routines. Without supervision you might see a pattern emerge that wouldn't surprise a neuroscientist – the brain loves patterns – but will probably surprise you. Many families are taken aback to find that a child has been operating on a regular pattern, but one cycling at twenty-five or twenty-six hours instead of twenty-four. This meant they were actually following the child's pattern around the clock, allowing the child to stay up later and later at night, and getting up with them one or two hours later each morning. As a result, at times family members had to get extra sleep during the day. Of course, the child was just operating on a normal circadian rhythm, but this needed to be reset to twenty-four hours each day.

While irregular schedules and biological rhythms may be the key factors affecting children's sleep, these disturbances are often complicated by **other problems** we've looked at elsewhere. If the child is not tired when you want them to go to sleep, you may be accidentally teaching them to **associate** being rocked or having a bottle with you trying to put them down, which may mean they are unable to get back to sleep after normal night-time wakings. (See **Building good associations for *excellent sleep*** on pages 160 to 171.) If you're not firm enough at bedtime, they may always stay up too late, and the time at which they're able to get to sleep may shift.

Helping them may involve several factors. When they have sleep problems involving a disturbance in their rhythms, it will not be enough simply to correct their sleep associations or to be firmer. You'll need to correct their schedule as well, by learning to understand their particular schedule disruptors.

Even if their schedule is perfectly regular, these routines can be problematic if they are poorly timed. In this case, a number of subtler factors can influence sleep, with the result that the child may have **problems getting to sleep** or **wake too early in the morning**.

Problems getting to sleep

When it comes to bedtime difficulties, we have already discussed many causes. But there are **three other, schedule-related causes** of inability to sleep at bedtime that affect children, despite a regular schedule. These are:

1. a **late sleep phase**

2. an **inappropriately late bedtime**

3. problems relating to **naps**

If your child never seems tired at bedtime and you have looked at all the other possibilities discussed in this book, it could be that they are an **'owl'**. They will be at their best late in the evening and always have trouble waking in the morning, no matter how much sleep they get. They may have difficulty falling asleep at the proper time.

A late sleep phase is common in adults, but happens less often with children, who in fact fall asleep far more easily. If your child has a tendency to be wide awake near bedtime, you should still be able to avoid major problems as long as you keep them on a regular schedule. Make sure they wake up at the same time every day, and plan ahead to ensure an unrushed bedtime routine. We'll look at this problem in more detail later.

If your child seems **very sleepy a while before you put them to bed**, you are probably waiting too long. Try an earlier bedtime with a nice bedtime ritual and they will fall asleep relatively quickly.

Late-afternoon naps, **too many naps** and **not enough naps** all have high impacts on children's sleep–wake patterns, and certainly on bedtime difficulties.

Waking too early

If your child is waking too early, there are two brain-based possibilities. One is caused by an **early sleep phase**, in which your child falls asleep and wakes too early. Dealing with early risers – what we often call **'larks'** – is a tricky business. Many children do not respond, despite all our efforts, because they wake up early feeling alert and active. Early morning is their best time and they tire and run out of steam in the evening. We'll look at this in more detail on page 195. As we saw in **Part 2**, the same occurs with adults, but they tend to be more bothered by a tendency to stay up late at night than by getting up early.

Children can also wake too early when they have a **short sleep requirement**: they actually need less sleep than you think they do, and wake early for this reason. But don't be too quick to see this as the solution. Even if you make bedtime later, you may find they continue to wake early. It's quite possible they have learned to **associate** something with waking at that time, such as light in the room or noise from outside.

Before deciding that they need less sleep, see if they sleep longer in the morning if you keep their room dark. Try postponing your response to them a little more each day to give them a chance to sleep a little longer. Use the **association** techniques we went through earlier (pages 160 to 171). Practise these for a few weeks in the hope of getting your child to do one additional sleep cycle each night.

Lifestyle clashes

Sometimes we are dissatisfied with our child's sleep patterns but they are in fact **completely normal**. The patterns simply don't work well with our lifestyle. Some patterns are very irritating to us. We need to be mindful that children only need a certain amount of sleep, and we will have to consider *their* schedule as well as *our own*. Most children cannot sleep fifteen hours a day. If they are sleeping up to twelve hours at night, this is quite normal. It is **our expectations** that need to be adjusted.

You can't have it both ways, putting them to bed early and waking them up late. But you can **adjust their schedule** so it's more in line with your own. Watch how much sleep they get, then adjust their present sleep period so that it better fits with your schedule. Unfortunately, you will probably have to make concessions, by being up with them later at night or getting up earlier in the morning.

Normal, early and late sleep phases

Like adults, children have sleep–wake rhythms that are **closely synchronised** with their **other body rhythms**, and especially with changes to their **body temperature**. If we try to put them to bed in the waking phase, when their body temperature is high, they will simply not be sleepy. If we try to wake them during the sleep phase, when their body temperature is still low, they will be unwilling to wake.

Many children – infants, toddlers, primary-school-aged children and adolescents – show a preference for either **early mornings** or **late evenings**. It's not known at what age children develop these sleep-phase differences, and how often they carry them into adulthood. It is also unclear whether these differences are genetic, or arise from environmental factors.

Early sleep phases

Early sleep phases – falling asleep and waking up far earlier than desired – occur often enough to be problematic, especially in very young children. It's easy to recognise this problem and correct it, but it requires a little time. It can take up to **two weeks** to shift the sleep rhythms by as little as **one to two hours**. You have to look at the child's total daily schedule, not just the bedtime one. You may need to alter nap times and mealtimes and make some other compromises. If they are already getting the sleep they need, you'll need to change the time of day they sleep, knowing you can't increase the hours. Where do want their sleep phase to be? If you want them to wake later, then this means later bedtimes.

Late sleep phases

The late sleep phase also commonly afflicts children of all ages. Children will experience difficulty falling asleep at the expected bedtime, **regardless of bedtime rituals or punishments**. They will also have difficulty waking at a normal time. You will find there are no struggles or sleep problems when they *are* allowed to go to bed later than the usual time. And if they suffer *only* from a late sleep phase, there will be **no night-time waking up**.

Many parents get quite upset when dealing with this issue. They become confused and concerned, particularly by the child's behaviours and the lack of success they have with trying to get the child to sleep and wake up earlier. At first they feel they're being too soft, and so they refuse to give in to the child. They often punish the child's 'failures' by removing privileges and occasionally with spankings. All of this, of course, only makes matters worse.

The natural impulse at this stage is to think there must really be something wrong with the child, but this is almost never the case. The fact is **they will go to sleep when they are ready to sleep**. Spending multiple hours lying in bed, tossing, turning and over-thinking, unable to fall asleep, is very unpleasant. For many children, if they're wide awake, alone, in a dark room with no distractions, it will lead to scary fantasies in bed. It's not surprising that they vehemently object to going to bed early. The dilemma they are faced with every night is **whether to suffer alone in bed, or get up and make their parents angry**.

How does a late sleep phase begin? There are a number of causes, but the most common is **the natural tendency of the sleep cycle to drift later** unless held in check by a regular and appropriate schedule. If your child **doesn't have a regular schedule** and is allowed to stay up late and sleep in, the cycle will gradually drift on its own. If they go through a period in which **temporary fears, excitement or an illness** interfere with falling asleep, and they are also allowed to sleep late, their cycle is likely to shift. Even when conditions return to normal, they will experience problems falling asleep and waking up at the times they did previously.

Family patterns are most definitely important in determining late phase development. If you like to sleep late,

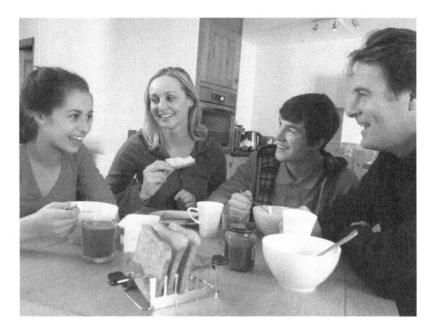

and are happy if your child sleeps late, the temptation is to wake them regularly at a later time, causing their sleep phase to begin to shift. If you are an early riser and are unwilling to sit around waiting for them to wake up on their own, it is less likely that their sleep phase will become delayed.

So how do you **solve** this problem? When you're sure the issue is a late sleep phase, and your child has not reached the **teen years**, the solution is fairly straightforward. Start with a schedule that fits their present times of falling asleep and waking up, then introduce gradual increases in the sleep phase by **making their bedtime and waking time a little earlier each day**.

Allow them (for now) to stay up until about the time they normally fall asleep, so that you can be assured they will fall asleep easily. This should make bedtime pleasant and free of tension, bickering, anxiety and frustration. If they are old enough to understand, they will be relieved to know you are no longer angry with them for not settling down earlier, and that you now accept their being allowed to stay up later.

You now have to decide **when you want them to go to sleep and wake up**. If you and your child do not have to be up and about early, you'll have quite a few options. But if there are caveats around bedtimes and wake-up times due to family circumstances or school, they will affect how much you can adjust the schedule.

To move the sleep phase earlier, you will need to begin **in the morning**. There is no way you can make a child fall asleep, but waking them up is something you *can* control. Begin with their natural waking-up time. **Every one or two days, wake them about fifteen minutes earlier**. Once you have reached the desired times, you may have to continue to advance the evening bedtime a little. It is hard to get this exactly right, so you may require some flexibility to ensure you attain the earlier sleep phase.

At this point you may have to make other small changes in sleep times and daily routines to ensure a sleep pattern that is both acceptable and workable. If your child's **nap times** and **mealtimes** are late, you will have to change these very gradually as you wind back their bedtime and getting-up times. This process does mean that they will be a little more tired during the day and want to start napping for fifteen to twenty minutes longer. But you'll need to make sure you don't allow this to happen. If they have been napping for an hour and twenty minutes, **hold them to that schedule** so that they go to bed a little earlier at night.

You will know that your child's late sleep phase problem is improving when they begin to **wake on their own at the right time in the morning**, especially when they get up for **school**. This is a significant sign that their sleep phase is in the right place in the twenty-four-hour day.

*

Finally, let's look at **adolescents**, who often have problems with late sleep phase. Most love to stay up late with their **digital devices**, if not talking to their friends then playing games or listening to music. **Pressure** from peers to conform is very strong. On weekends in particular, teenagers frequently stay up late then sleep until midday or later, and their sleep cycles can move around significantly. As a result, they may be very sleep-deprived during the week when they actually need to be at their best (a bit like the students in my sleep class).

Adolescents with a late sleep phase are harder to help than younger children, because **it is far more difficult for parents or carers to assume control over an adolescent's sleep cycles**. Even if the teenager understands the importance of maintaining a regular sleep schedule, they may be unwilling to go along with the proposed changes.

Theoretically, they could change their very late sleep phase by **getting up early seven days a week and having no naps during the day**. However, in practice, such a five- or six-hour shift would be very difficult for a fifteen-year-old to achieve. All the time they were shifting, they would be getting

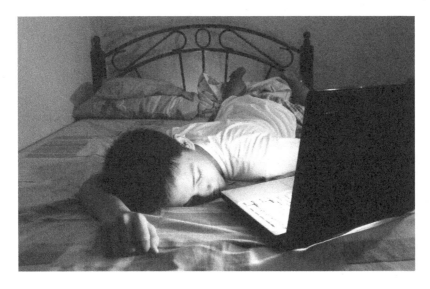

much less sleep than they needed. They would be tired, their motivation would drop and they would probably go back to sleeping late on weekends. (The only way this method works well is if their sleep phase is **only slightly late** – see the next page for details.)

A different approach would be for them not to rely on parents or carers and in effect to **take over the role of solving the problem for themselves**. They should be responsible for getting up in the morning – for example, making sure a loud wake-up alarm is set, with the snooze button turned off. They will also need to make the decision to stop using devices, listening to the radio and so on when it is time to go to sleep. Although doing these things before bed may be more pleasurable than just lying quietly, the fact is that their brain will continue processing what they have been looking at or listening to, such as radio chatter, and make it harder for them to fall asleep.

The easiest and quickest way for a teenager to correct their late sleep phase is in fact **to go to bed later each night**. Instead of struggling to get to sleep earlier, they delay their bedtime by **at least three hours each night** and get up **three hours later each day**, until they have gone around the clock to the time wanted. This schedule follows our natural tendency to stay up and wake up a little later each day.

For example, the first night they go to sleep at 7am and plan to wake at 3pm. The next day, bedtime is 10am and they get up at 6pm. This pattern of continual and progressive change goes on until they arrive at an appropriate sleep schedule. If they oversleep during this process, it can be helpful to speed it up, but once they are near the correct times it is very important for them not to sleep past 6.30am.

During this period of adjustment, they will miss one or two days of school, but they can keep the time missed to a minimum by starting the change in **the early hours of a**

Saturday morning. If they do this, they will be sleeping during the mornings of Saturday, Sunday and Monday, while on Tuesday and Wednesday they won't be going to sleep until after school. During this period they will learn to fall asleep quickly, get enough sleep and not have much difficulty waking up. They should lose any unpleasant feelings they have learned to associate with bed.

Within **a week** they should be waking and sleeping at the desired times. As long as they keep their morning waking times constant, their sleep cycle will remain regular and will be progressively more stable. Once their sleep schedule is adjusted, you should find they are attending school far more punctually than before.

If the teenager's sleep phase is only **one and a half to three hours late**, it may make more sense to try to correct the phase shift by **starting with a late bedtime and moving it progressively earlier**, while **keeping the time of waking early** every day and **avoiding any naps**. Again, this is something you can't do for them. You can explain the why and how, but *they* must want to change and be prepared to get themselves up in the mornings.

However, there are some teenagers who **actually *want* a late sleep phase but are not prepared to admit it**. If this is the case, then the recommendations just described will not work. For some there can be no direct solution, because the late sleep phase is not the problem. It's only a **symptom of other, emotional problems** that may need professional help.

Teenagers must want to change their sleep patterns and be prepared to get themselves up in the mornings.

It is critical to understand what is causing their poor sleep before trying to correct what you *perceive* to be the problem. **When the *real* issues are isolated and understood, sleep problems will usually resolve themselves** without the need for carefully planned schedule changes. Adjustments to sleep schedules may still be required, but this can occur after the source of the problem has been identified.

Monitoring sleep debt

One of the least obvious of sleep problems is lost sleep, or what is commonly called 'sleep debt'. There is no absolute way of measuring whether the amount you or your child sleep per day is appropriate. A child who is not getting enough sleep may **wake repeatedly during the night**, as well as, or instead of, having **bedtime struggles**. If they don't have these issues, you can watch their **behaviour** closely during the day to see whether they seem excessively sleepy or cranky. But the symptoms of insufficient sleep can often be very subtle.

If your two-year-old sleeps only **eight hours** at night (instead of the **twelve to fourteen hours** recommended on page 15) but seems to be happy and functioning well during the day, it may be tempting to assume they have no need for more sleep. But eight hours is rarely enough for a child of that age, and with proper intervention they can learn to increase their sleep time considerably.

When that happens, you may begin to notice an improvement in their general behaviour. Only then will you be aware of the subtler indicators of sleep debt that were actually evident *before* you adjusted their sleep schedule. The outcomes will be a happier child in the daytime – less irritable, more able to concentrate at play, and less inclined to have tantrums, accidents and arguments.

As we saw in the previous section on sleep phases, **adolescents** often do not get enough sleep either, and it's primarily a late sleep phase that needs adjusting. Teenagers are not likely to wake spontaneously on school days and tend to sleep at least one hour longer on weekends. When adolescents have the opportunity to sleep as much as they like, they will average about **nine hours** per night, and this is about the optimal level for their age (see the table on page 15).

THE VITAL MISSING HOUR

I've focused on some of the significant issues that adults and parents confront when dealing with children who sleep poorly. But it's also important to note that many children who do not experience these issues may still be suffering from lack of sleep, while managing to fly under the radar.

In recent National Sleep Foundation surveys, 90 per cent of parents believed their children were getting enough sleep. However, more than 60 per cent of the children surveyed reported extreme daytime sleepiness, and a quarter felt their academic performance had declined as a result. Nearly a quarter of that group had fallen asleep in class during the previous week.

The National Sleep Foundation research shows that half of all adolescents sleep less than seven hours a night during the school week, and by the time they reach senior secondary school they average only six and a half hours of sleep per night. The most striking statistic here is that only 5 per cent of senior students average eight hours a night. Some recent major studies show that from primary school through to secondary school children get around one hour less sleep each night than thirty years ago.

Adults who are reading this will already be churning through the reasons: too many things to do in a day; too much homework; late bedtimes; televisions, computers and other devices in bedrooms. But adults also contribute to the problem by coming home late themselves, and by wanting to be with

continued

the children but not wanting to be the one who tells them to go to bed.

It's only recently that sleep scientists have been able to measure the impact of this one hour of lost sleep on health. Children's and young adults' brains develop fast up to the age of twenty-one and much of that development occurs while they are asleep. There is now significant evidence that a lack of sleep could be associated with many illnesses and conditions that are common among young people, including obesity and ADHD (attention deficit hyperactivity disorder).

Functional MRI scans allow us to better understand the effects of sleep loss on brain function. Teachers and parents often note how difficult it is for children who are tired to learn and remember what they are taught. Scans show that it is because the neurons in their brain function poorly due to lost plasticity and they become incapable of making the synaptic connections necessary to create memories.

As explained earlier (pages 9 to 10), during sleep the brain is very busy with many processes that are critical to our functioning. Notably, it shifts what it has learned during the day from its memory-holding tank, the hippocampus, to other parts of the brain for storage; organises thoughts, analyses outcomes and sets goals; and extracts glucose from the bloodstream to provide energy for these processes. The more we have learned during the day, the longer we need to sleep for all of this to happen. Insufficient sleep means the brain will not have time to store all that has been learned or maintain adequate energy levels. In the classroom, loss of sleep often manifests as inattention, poor impulse control and diversion-seeking.

The amount of learning our children have to do each day is steadily increasing. Yet the sleep time they require to allow them to process this information is declining. Despite all the evidence, we adults and parents often feel that enforcing another hour of sleep for our children is not feasible. Or we regard sleep as a reflection of character, rather than a physical need, and consider fatigue a sign of weakness. We have put up with poor sleep for years and managed to cope with it, we say to ourselves.

But our children's developing brains are another story. Our children are simply not getting enough sleep and we should do everything in our power to give them that extra hour science shows they need.

LIGHTS OUT:
TIME TO SLEEP BETTER
THAN YOU EVER
HAVE BEFORE

'I love to sleep. Do you? Isn't it great?
It really is the best of both worlds.
You get to be alive and unconscious.'

—Rita Rudner, American comedian (1953–)

The goal of neuroscience is to help us improve all aspects of our lives. This includes improving what we know about sleep and, more importantly, improving *how* we sleep.

Our understanding of this critical aspect of our daily lives is constantly expanding as neurological technologies are improved. And these technologies are making us ask just as many questions as they answer. But that has always been the nature of science. And it means that in the future our knowledge of sleep will only get better.

I started this book talking about those undergraduate students who couldn't even tell me how much sleep they'd

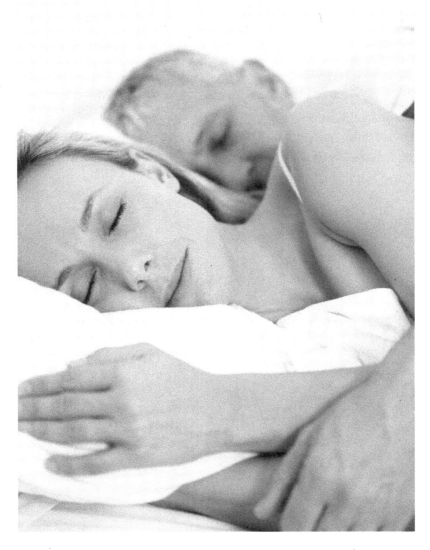

had the night before. Like so many of us, they lacked a proper understanding of what sleep does for our brains and bodies, and why getting enough of it is so critical.

In this book I've tried to give you that understanding. I've shown you what is going on in the brain during sleep, and how that can be improved for each one of us. I've also tried to encourage you to see sleep as more than just something that gets our attention when things go wrong.

We all experience sleep problems from time to time, and for some of us they're more frequent. The main issue, though, is not 'Do I have a *sleep problem?*' but 'How can I *sleep better?*'

We all need to be proactive, not just at night but during the day too. We need to be actively working towards having better sleep, more often, and eventually *all the time* (which is what I would call *excellent sleep*). Why? Because the better we sleep, the better we perform – mentally, physically and spiritually. Time to turn off the lights and have an *excellent sleep.*

Also by Stan Rodski

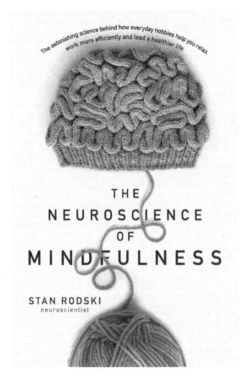

Cutting-edge studies in neuroscience have in recent years proved what many doctors, therapists and other health professionals had long suspected: simple, repetitive tasks, performed with focus and attention – mindfulness, in other words – can not only quieten our noisy thought processes and help us relax but also improve our outlook on life and protect us against a range of life-threatening illnesses.

A cognitive neuroscientist and a leading authority on mental performance, Stan Rodski sets out the science behind these remarkable discoveries in simple terms, and explains how you in turn can benefit from them. As well as examining the potentially pivotal role of mindfulness in alleviating stress and managing energy, Stan highlights the most effective mindfulness activities, guides you through quick and easy exercises, and shows you how to harness the power of mindfulness over the long term to forge mental and physical resilience – and create a happier, healthier, more compelling future.

More mindfulness tools from Stan Rodski

Colourtation – *the New Meditation*

The simple act of colouring has the power to reduce stress, improve mood and kindle creativity by creating new neural pathways and connections in our brains. Stan Rodski's *Colourtation* series spawned a colouring-book boom and was included in Oprah Winfrey's 2016 Christmas Wish List.

'Filling in the blanks has become one of my preferred ways to de-stress. Who knew? Besides being just plain fun, these three [books] will help with mental agility, focus and inner peace.' Oprah Winfrey

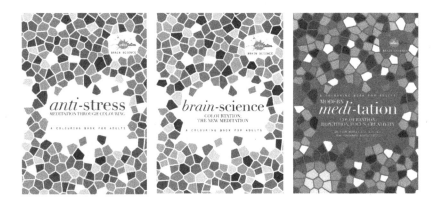

Available at all good bookstores and at www.colourtation.com

Anti-Stress *colouring books*

The designs in these six colouring books are based on Stan Rodski's research into neuroscience, particularly the beneficial effects of using repetition, pattern and control to quickly relax the brain. Offering fascinating insights into how we can better understand and improve our brain health, the series also looks at how colour affects our feelings, how to stimulate the brain, our fight-or-flight response, the science of focus and attention, and how to improve our thinking agility and resilience.

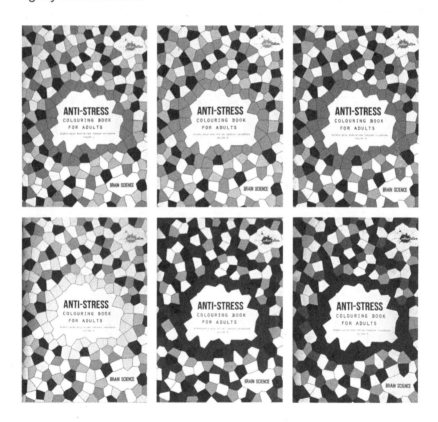

Available at www.colourtation.com